Becoming lean and fit is not a matter of training for a few weeks, like Rocky, to become a world champion. That only happens in Hollywood movies that portray professional athletes exercising for hours every day until they're exhausted. Real athletes never do that. They train only to the point that they can recover for the next day's training. Their progress comes in small increments, not heroic triumphs. Unfortunately, movies have persuaded people that they can become lean and fit virtually overnight. Even the weight loss and fitness industry bought into this distortion and began pushing people to become like Rocky. When that approach failed, because people were injuring themselves or burning out or jumping from one program to another, trainers began to entertain their clients instead of finding solutions to their problems. If you want to become truly lean and fit, you must work at it like an athlete, following a structured routine—and that is easier and more pleasant than you may expect.

The principles that work for athletes also work for ordinary people of all ages. Athletes, of course, have coaches. The Happy Body program, on the other hand, will teach you everything you need to know to be your own coach. This innovative program establishes, for the first time, exact scientific and testable methods and goals to engineer your own weight loss and fitness within precise time periods. That empowers you to self-correct your progress at every step.

The Happy Body is a total health program, not just an exercise or diet plan. It will teach you to safely lose 1.0 to 2.5 pounds every week, and keep them off, without getting stuck at plateaus. You will have full control over the process, right down to the ounce.

In addition to teaching you how to lose weight, the program will also help you to restore the flexibility and posture you had as a young child, and to be leaner, stronger, and faster than you have ever been. In essence, The Happy Body program will not only make you as youthful as you were at twenty, but twenty as you would have been if you had followed the program at that age.

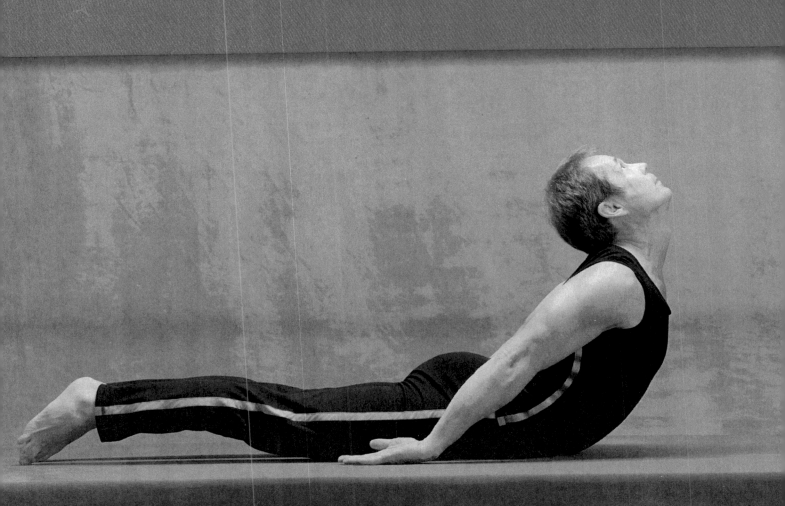

THE HAPPY BODY

ANIELA & JERZY GREGOREK

PHOTOGRAPHY BY JEFF BOXER AND JEFF SARPA
BOOK DESIGN BY ALEXANDER ATKINS DESIGN, INC.

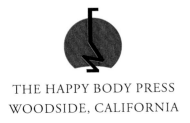

THE HAPPY BODY PRESS
WOODSIDE, CALIFORNIA

The Happy Body Press, P.O. Box 620901, Woodside, California 94062
Second Edition

The authors advise readers to take full responsibility for their safety and well-being. Before beginning the diet and/or exercises described in this book, be sure that you do not take risks beyond your level of ability and comfort. As with any diet or exercise program, talk with your physician about whether this program is safe and right for you.

Gregorek, Aniela & Jerzy
The happy body: the simple science of nutrition, exercise, and relaxation
Aniela & Jerzy Gregorek
ISBN-13: 978-0-9962439-2-6
ISBN-10: 0996243925

To learn more about The Happy Body program visit www.thehappybody.com.

Cover & interior design: Alexander Atkins Design, Inc. [alexatkinsdesign.com]
Gym and Zen photography: Jeff Boxer [jeffboxer.com]; Makeup: Kerry Herta
Food photography: Jeff Sarpa [jeffsarpa.com]; Food styling: Diane Elander [dianeelander.com]
Tableware provided by Heath Ceramics [heathceramics.com] and Luna Garcia [lunagarcia.com]

We dedicate this book to all our coaches and clients, and to our greatest teacher— our daughter, Natalie.

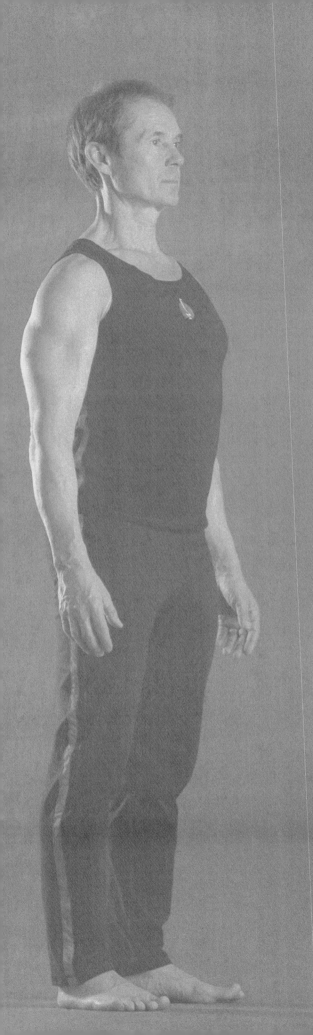

The Philosophy of The Happy Body

Part 1

Part 2

Designing Your Happy Body

TESTIMONIALS

Nourishing Your Happy Body

Part 3

FOREWORD

We asked three health professionals who practice The Happy Body to write about the program from their unique perspectives: The medical benefits of the program are presented by physician, Dr. Eric Weiss; the skeletomuscular benefits are described by kinesiologist, Professor Stuart McGill, and the psychological benefits are outlined by psychologist, Judith Hecker, Ph.D.

Getting Off Your Medications

ERIC L. WEISS, MD

Founder & CEO, The Village Doctor; Associate Clinical Professor, Stanford University School of Medicine

Youth is wasted on the young, my father used to say. And as we all age, we know exactly what he meant. As a physician, I see many patients who feel much older than their chronological age. Why is this? Often it is because the habits and routines of years ago have faded and been replaced by hours of inactivity punctuated by business lunches, stressful meetings, and overscheduled days. What follows are body changes we can all see from the outside: extra pounds, lack of fitness, and poor posture. But even more important are the changes that can be measured on the inside: elevated blood cholesterol and blood sugar, insulin resistance, and high blood pressure. These patients already feel bad enough without medications, and then their alertness, athleticism, and libido become subject to the side effects of the drugs used to treat what are now chronic medical problems. These drugs include statins for cholesterol control, diabetes medications for blood sugar control, and an array of others to control blood pressure.

Neither the patients nor the physicians are happy with these changes, and many discussions occur in doctors' offices across the country regarding diet and exercise. Diet books are read and personal trainers are hired, but almost always, over time, the "old" bodies return. This is because the fundamental relationship with diet and exercise has not changed. Almost by definition, diets require sacrifice—of both quantity and quality of food. Exercise becomes a means to an end, with patients slogging through 30-minute sessions on a Stairmaster or grinding through 2-mile runs. Both the diet and the exercise are joyless and hence never become habitual, much less ritual. I would argue that people believe that good health is all about losing weight. That is essential, but how it is done is more important. Their goal should be to look forward to their exercise and to change their relationship with food. Youth-promoting exercise can be joyful, and healthy meals can be delicious.

I learned this about two years ago, when I noticed that some of my patients were dramatically losing weight and becoming healthier—and, in fact, their whole outlook on life seemed to be changing for the better. When I asked them what they were doing differently, they all mentioned The Happy Body program.

Their changes were so impressive that I decided to try the program and see for myself why it worked so well. Even though I was in good physical shape, I got even better—and fast.

Since then, I have had the pleasure of referring my most knowledgeable but frustrated patients to Jerzy and Aniela's Happy Body program, and the results have been astounding. Not only have my patients lost pounds, but they have also redesigned their bodies so that they have achieved a desirable proportion of weight to height and muscle to fat. Furthermore, patients who used to have dangerous levels of blood pressure, cholesterol, and sugar, which required prescription medications for control, are now off all their medications and only take a few supplements with a preventive medicine focus. But what impresses me most are the mental changes I have seen: alertness, better sleep, more energy, and return of libido. In addition, patients find a whole new relationship with their food. Yogurt is more desirable to them than chocolate chip cookies, and even tastier. Whole grain breads are more satisfying than french fries. Cooking in the kitchen with a spouse or friend is more creative and fun than going out.

The exercises in The Happy Body program artfully combine the benefits of weightlifting, yoga, and Pilates. The diet in the program combines an emphasis on organic vegetables and lean proteins with a schedule to optimize metabolism. Most important, Aniela and Jerzy recognize the role of meditation and "recovery" both to amplify the benefits of exercise and to balance out the stressors of daily life. Their diet, exercise, and recovery routine is not a chore but the best part of your day—not only a habit but a ritual, and as such, something you can enjoy for the rest of your life.

The Healthy Spine

STUART McGILL, PH.D.
Chair of the Department of Kinesiology, University of Waterloo, Canada

We all want a body that is robust, performs well, and is impervious to injury—in summary, a "happy" body. Achieving a happy body requires wisdom together with the discipline to execute a plan. In today's society, despite all the research and "knowledge growth," finding the wisdom to create a happy body is unfortunately rare. So-called fitness experts encourage long-distance running or bodybuilding workout programs, both of which are ill-suited for most people, who usually become sore and injured in the process and then quit.

My friends Jerzy and Aniela Gregorek are both highly accomplished athletes and coaches, who have attained valuable wisdom through decades of world-class competition in weightlifting. In this book, they have refined that wisdom down to its essential principles. By mastering these, readers will be able to assess their own bodies and select the proper approach to make them "happy." The knowledge contained in these pages is true to science, untainted by any commercial agendas.

The Happy Body exercises, combined with relaxation techniques, are designed not only to naturally balance and build joints but also to correct movement flaws that, over time, have already resulted in joint damage. All this, coupled with nutritional wisdom, leads to performance that most people think was lost with their youth.

In all my years as a professor of spine biomechanics, I have conducted countless experiments in my search for the wisdom that is needed to attain health, avoid injury, and enhance performance. My journey would have been simpler had I read The Happy Body years ago.

Happy Body, Happy Mind

Judith Hecker, Ph.D.
Psychologist, Los Angeles, California

Aniela and Jerzy, my good friends and coaches, asked me to write about the psychological aspects of training with The Happy Body method. I am a clinical psychologist practicing in Los Angeles and a faculty member of the California Graduate Institute in Pacifica and the Geffen School of Medicine at UCLA. The following remarks are based on my observations of the psychological changes that have accompanied the physical changes both in myself and in my friends who practice The Happy Body program.

First, about maintaining a sense of control in tough times: These comments are written in October 2008, during a period of economic turmoil and recession. We have all become painfully aware that we are not in control of the value of our houses, the stability of our jobs, or the security of our finances. There is, however, one area in which we can maintain control in the face of chaos: namely, our own bodies. We can go into a quiet room and work out. The weightlifting workout of The Happy Body program demands total focus. We have to concentrate on correct movement, breathing, and balance. During the time we train, we have to follow a precise plan, so for the duration of the workout, it is nearly impossible to think about the loss of control outside. And once the workout is over, the sense of focus and of having exercised some measure of control during our day continues to support us.

Second, about fostering a sense of calmness: We are often overwhelmed by spreading our lives too thin and taking on too many obligations. This leads to health, relational, and family problems that we cannot resolve. Taking half an hour out of every day to do our workout gives us the mental space to calm down and reorient ourselves. As we follow the workouts over time, we start to feel less irritable with our lives, and other people tell us that we have become more pleasant and much calmer. Third, about benefiting from routines: In the United States, advertising and marketing have led us to believe that what is new is always improved, that change is always better. We therefore look for the latest exercise method, the newest fitness gadgets, the most recent diet fad. We do not realize the value of doing the same set of exercises, day after day. Yet in ancient exercise systems, such as tai-chi and yoga, there is a keen awareness of the physical and mental benefits of precisely following the same daily routine. For a pianist, a master craftsman, or a mystic, there is no doubt about the benefits of repeating the same exercises over and over.

The routine that is set out in this book works like a mantra in meditation. It will clear your mind and make it easier for you to deal with the stresses in your life.

PREFACE

When Jerzy was weightlifting in Poland at the age of 16, he was impatient to improve his performance. At that time, the latest fad in conditioning was long-distance running. So Jerzy got up early every morning and was out the door by 6:00, running through the forest near his house.

One day, after Jerzy had been running for three months, his coach, Andrzej Kowalczyk, approached him in the gym, looking concerned.

"Why are you so slow?" he asked.

Jerzy was surprised because he thought he was doing fine.

"Is everything alright at home?" the coach asked.

"Yes, everything's fine."

"What about school?"

"Fine."

"What time do you go to bed at night?"

"Ten."

"Okay, tell me everything you do during the day, hour by hour."

"Well, I wake up at 5:45 and run through the forest for one hour."

"Did I tell you to run?"

"No."

"So, why do you run?"

"I thought it would make me a better weightlifter. Faster."

"So, what do you think? Wouldn't I know whether you should run or not?"

"Yeah, I guess you would."

"Okay, listen carefully, because I'm only going to tell you this once. You need to learn to keep your body happy."

Jerzy laughed. But seeing that his coach was serious, he stopped, feeling awkward.

"If you keep your body happy," the coach continued, "it means you wake up in the morning and you look forward to the day, eager to do everything. If you don't keep your body happy, you gradually start to fear the day. Then you wake up feeling tired and overwhelmed. Some of the things you want to do seem too much, so you start making excuses not to do them. That's the first way to tell whether you're keeping your body happy or not."

"That explains," Jerzy said, "why I used to wake up before the clock rang, and now I wish I could sleep more."

"Now you know. That's the first sign. The second thing is to watch your performance. If thinking about breaking a record excites you, then you are doing fine. But if it frightens you, you are pushing yourself too hard. My job is to make sure that your body is happy by keeping you in that gap between doing too much and not enough. The better lifter you become, the narrower that gap will get. That's the test of how well you are mastering your craft."

Years later, when Jerzy and Aniela became coaches, they found themselves telling their clients that if they wanted to achieve strong, healthy, and youthful bodies—in short, if they wanted to have happy bodies—they had to pursue that like a professional athlete. There is a craft to becoming strong, healthy, and youthful, always calibrating what is too much and what is not enough. This book will guide you toward mastering that craft.

ACKNOWLEDGMENTS

T his book is a response to all the hundreds of people who have challenged and inspired us over the last twenty-five years to find solutions to their health and fitness problems. We can't name them all, but here are some who had the greatest impact on The Happy Body program:

First of all, we thank our Olympic weightlifting coaches, Andrzej Kowalczyk and Waldemar Baszanowski, for teaching us proper technique and the discipline and patience to achieve it.

Thanks to Charlie Henderson, 80-year-old master weightlifter, whose greatness inspired us to discover our Standard of Strength and for all people.

We also thank all our long-lasting clients who have become our friends and supporters over the years, especially: Tony Abbis; Kathy Adzich; Cie Marie & David Anderson; Laura Jean & Jim Anderson; Lisett & Karl Angel; Ralph Angel; Veronica Arthur; Jennifer J. Bailey; Robert Baldwin; Sybilla & Alex Balkanski; Lorna Basso; Patrick Bujold; Mayur Baugh; Barrance Baytos; Susan Bockus; Carolyn Bowsher; Gilda Brasch; Anitha Brown; Andrew, Lauren & Susan Buchanan; Raquel E. Burgos; Andrea Campbell; Kelly Carter; Michael Casey; Walter Chi; Bud Coligan; Wendy Cook; Simone Otus Coxe; Colette & Kim Cranston; Ellen Curry; Jon Curry; Peggy Dalal; Kristal Dehnad; Peggy & Steve Dow; Samantha Dinsmore; Kelly Dozois; Cathleen Edidin; Haleh Endrissi; Stacey Escobar, Kimberly Essen; Light & Summer Eternity; Fran Evans; Pam & Jim Everett; Bob Falkenberg; Acenia, Toby, Casey & Caleb Farrand; Barbara & Billy Finkelstein; Karen Fisher; Nanci, Gary, Leah & Josh Fredkin; Susan Friedman; Gwen Fuller; Gaurav Garg; Robert Garland; Tom Gately; Michelle A. Gerber; Ritu Ghumman; Dianne G. Giancarlo; Kelly & Greg Golub; Mark Gordon; Stacy Grant; Judith Greenberg; Nancy Greenbach; Martin & Ruth Gruber; Rick & Sandy Hahamian; Crystal Hayling; Malora Hardin; Teri Hausman; David Heart; Judy Hecker; Angela & George Hensler; Judy Heyboer; Chris Huntley; Susan & Joel Hyatt; Staphanie Ingster; Gildard Jackson; Suzanne & Sabrina Jain; Linda & Robert Jameson; Sigrid Jenson; Barry L. Johnson; Janis Kanter; Steven F. Kanter; Richard Kasznow; Jane & Mari Kawasaki; Michelle & David E. Kelley; Judy Kiel; Anne Kiser; Sheryl Klein; Fitnete Kraja; Jody Kramer; Erica Lapacka; Sharon Lebherz; E. J. "Doc" Kreis; Craig Liebenson; Peter Levitt; Aaron Lipsey; Alheli and Sabrina Maahs; Paul Mason; Debra Matiyahu; Eva Mees; Jamis MacNiven; Terry & Joe McClintock; Cheryl McCoy; Stuart McGill; Susan, Bridget & John Meaney; Chris Meledandri; Faye Mellos; Jean & Stephen Mereu; Ilona Merli; Carol J. Middleton; Annie & Bob Miller; Susan & John Mimi; Kris Moore; Christopher Morace; Mary Lynn Moran; Devon Morehead; Susan, Gib & Drew Myers; Jennifer Nash; Lori Nawn; William & Christy Neidig; James Nicholas; Linda, Guy, Brittney & Camille Nora;

Donna Novitsky; Inessa Obenhuber; Joyce Pacificar; Lisa R. Pieper; Amy Pietz; Catherine Pilibos; Francis Pinto; Barbara Pivnicka; Karen Plastiras; Tracy & Greg Plowman; Buffy Poon; Malgosia & Marek Probosz; John Quinn; Michele Raffin; Robyn Rajkovich; Saira Ramasastry; Dushanka Resenbaun; Michael Ricci; Bill, Pat, Billy and Don Robertson; Heidi Roizen; Liz Rome; Debbie & Stuart Rosenberg; Dusanka Rosenbaum; Debbie, Catherine, Amelia & Tom Rosch; Loren Lebherz, Sack; Nancy Savage; Helen S. Scheffler; Peter E. Schwab; Terry Sculley; Richard S. Seiler; Komal Shah; Jane Sharninghouse; Catherine Shaw; Metta Shields; Katie & J. D. Simpson; Carol L. Spence; Vijayashree Srinivasan; Liz Stangle; Barbara Stefik; Francine Swain; Betty & Roger Toguchi; Carol Torbett; Maddy & Jefffey Tucker; Christine VanDeVelde & Don Luskin; Phil Wagner; Pat & Rick Wallace; Kelly Walsh; Rey Walton James Warren; Cheryl Wayne; Tom Weary; Jessica Weisman; Eric & Jackie Weiss; Pam & Eugene Weiss; Helen & Maurice Werdegar; Janelle J. & Chris White; Mary White; Pat & Craig Whiteman; Nancy, Clark & Douglass Wigley; Reno & Coco Wilson; Amy and Arnold Wong; Jack & Lou Yeager; Patricia Yeh; John & Sylvia Vargas; Lisa Vidergauz; and Danielle Vontz.

Finally, we thank our photographers, Jeff Boxer and Jeff Sarpa, our copy editor Erin Barrett, and our graphic designer, Alexander Atkins.

THE PHILOSOPHY OF THE HAPPY BODY

PART 1

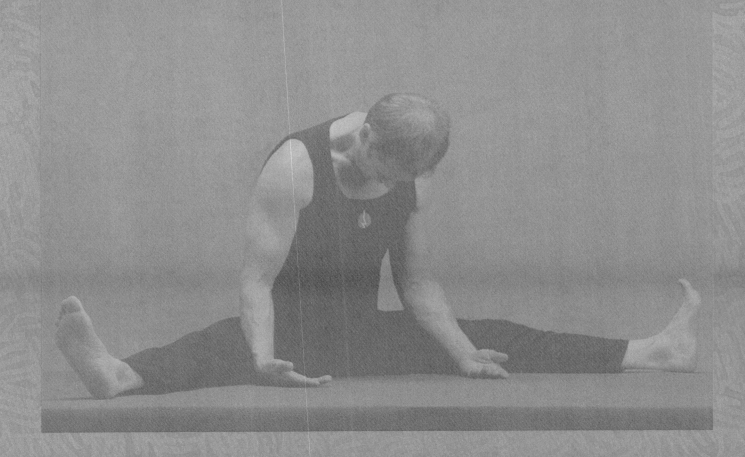

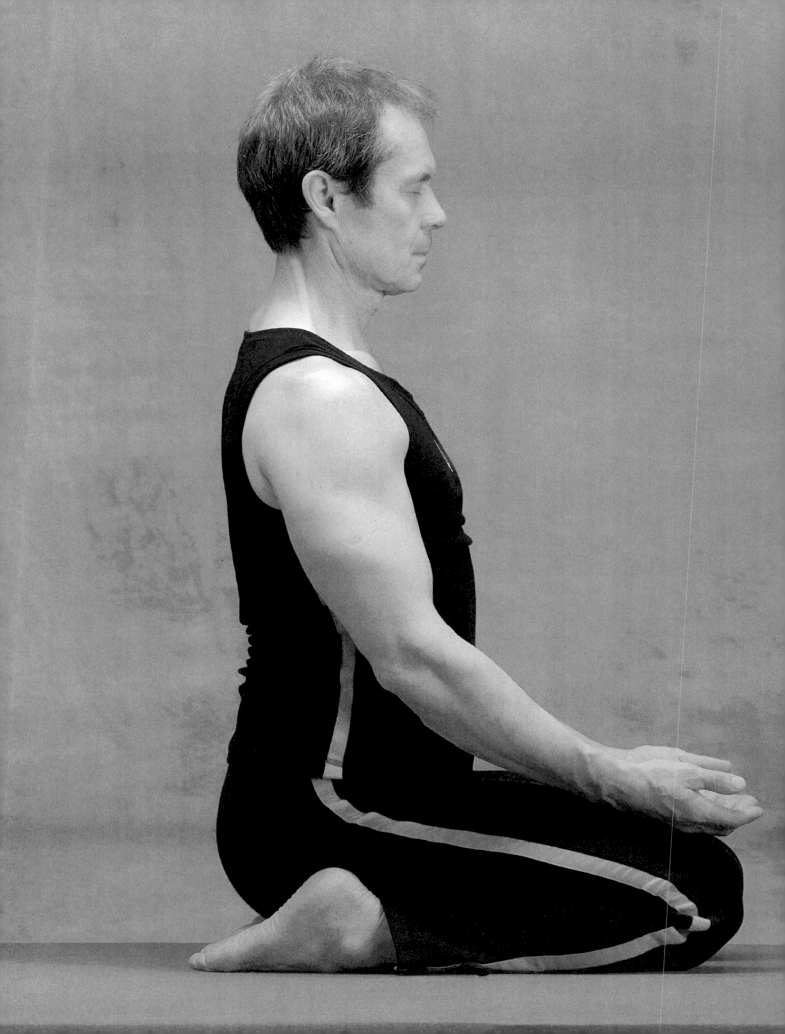

CHAPTER 1

Genesis of The Happy Body

YOUTHFULNESS

"All successful people have a goal. No one can get anywhere unless he knows where he wants to go and what he wants to be or do.
— NORMAN VINCENT PEALE

In our thirty years as weightlifting coaches, we have trained hundreds of people whose bodies have differed in capability and whose motivations have been diverse. Some were elite athletes who wanted to improve their performance; others had never trained before and wanted to regain lost functions, such as the ability to tie their shoes while standing, or to lift luggage without effort. Regardless of the words they used to explain why they wanted weightlifting coaching, we began to see a pattern in their motivations. Everyone wanted to regain—or in some cases, to have for the first time—the essential factors of youthfulness.

When we asked them to define youthfulness, most of them pointed to three principal qualities— high energy, agility, and good posture—and some added several others, including coordination, quickness, calmness, good looks, good health, and good sex.

But who has youthfulness, what are its components, and, most important, how can it be measured so that we can develop a plan to attain it?

WHO HAS YOUTHFULNESS?

Most people would answer that babies and children embody youthfulness. But babies and children only have some qualities of youthfulness, such as flexibility and high energy. They lack coordination and agility. The people who are truly youthful are athletes, especially those who must meet specific weight requirements, such as Olympic weightlifters, Olympic wrestlers, and judokas. They have all the good qualities that children have and more.

WHAT ARE THE COMPONENTS OF YOUTHFULNESS?

When we observed all athletes, we saw that some of them, such as sprinters, strive to increase speed; others, such as jumpers, strive to increase distance; and still others, such as weightlifters, strive to increase lifted weight. While only the sprinters work directly with speed, the other two work with it indirectly. Jumpers, for example, increase their jumping distance by increasing the speed of their impact with the ground, and weightlifters lift heavier weights by moving them faster. So one element common to all athletes is speed. However, speed cannot exist without flexibility and strength. If you are inflexible or weak, you will certainly be slow.

In terms of muscles, strength is the ability to contract, and flexibility, to expand. Fat, on the other hand, is excess baggage that doesn't help one to do either. In weightlifting, we say that fat doesn't lift. But we could also say that fat doesn't run, jump, or throw either. In other words, a lean body is more efficient than a fat one, so to increase your body's strength, flexibility, and speed, you must reduce your percentage of fat. However, efficiency does not only depend on that, but also on the relationship between height and weight. For example, sprinters cannot be too light or too heavy relative to their height, because either way they will lack the strength and speed to accelerate most efficiently. Thus, they must strive to achieve an ideal body weight.

There is one more quality that all athletes possess, and that is physical elegance—the beauty of their movement—which is made possible by good

THE SIX PRIMARY QUALITIES OF YOUTHFULNESS

1. Flexibility
2. Strength
3. Speed
4. Leanness
5. Ideal Body Weight
6. Good Posture

posture. If we were to watch them in slow motion, they would all look like dancers.

Thus, there are six primary qualities of youthfulness: 1. flexibility, 2. strength, 3. speed, 4. leanness, 5. ideal body weight, and 6. good posture.

The right combination of these qualities can only make an athlete better, but the ideal combination varies with each sport. For example, track-and-field athletes need to develop all six qualities to more or less the same degree. However, in football, a quarterback will principally train to increase his speed and agility, but a lineman will principally train to increase his strength and resistance to impact. There are also sports in which leanness is not required, such as sumo wrestling or shot put. Furthermore, some sports develop some parts of the body more than others. For example, sprinters develop muscles in their legs but not in their upper bodies.

There are also sports that develop all parts of the body equally and all six of the youthful qualities. These include baseball, basketball, figure skating, ice hockey, judo, Olympic weightlifting, Olympic wrestling, pole vaulting, rugby, swimming, volleyball, and water polo. Because these sports proportionately develop not only the body but also the six qualities of youthfulness, they are the most beneficial of all activities.

Athletes focus on what they do, not on how they look, although beauty comes along anyway.

Whether athletes run, throw, jump, hit, or lift, their success depends on the combination of the six primary qualities of youthfulness. However, the driving force behind these qualities is striving for goals. These vary somewhat, creating somewhat different bodies from sport to sport, because we become what we do. Thus, athletes focus on what they do, not on how they look, although beauty comes along anyway. They train from the inside out. Anyone else who wants to be youthful must focus, like athletes, on performance and movement, not on being beautiful.

Jumpers think all the time about jumping higher. Swimmers think about swimming faster. Weightlifters think about lifting greater weights. All athletes deal with numbers, whether directly or indirectly. They train to break records or win competitions. We marvel at their movement, which we may call poetry in motion as we admire sprinters racing down the track like cheetahs, figure skaters spinning on ice like tops, or pole vaulters flipping through the air like dolphins.

In the latter half of the twentieth century, coaches began to realize that they could not further improve their athletes' skills by just having them practice their sports. Olympic weightlifting develops the strongest and fastest of all athletic bodies, and weightlifters also have extremely flexible bodies, second only to gymnasts. Furthermore, weightlifters' movements—pulling, squatting, jumping, and throwing—are components of all other sports. For these reasons, coaches from other sports began to use weightlifting to improve their athletes' performance. Thus, sprinters, ice hockey players, gymnasts, football players, and other athletes have begun to train at the side of Olympic weightlifters. Today, almost every university in the United States has its athletes training in Olympic weightlifting to increase their strength, flexibility, and speed. At the UCLA Acosta Training Center, for example, there are fifty Olympic weightlifting platforms on which the best Bruin teams train.

BEING YOUR OWN YOUTHFULNESS COACH

The same principles that work for athletes also work for ordinary people of all ages. Athletes, of course, have coaches, but everyone else must be his or her own coach. The Happy Body program teaches you all you need to know to be your own coach. The program was designed to make the benefits of Olympic weightlifting accessible to the general population. It eliminates the complex and dangerous elements of weightlifting while establishing concrete standards as attainable goals of youthfulness for everyone. The Happy Body program will help you to restore the flexibility, ideal body weight, and posture you had as a young child, and to be leaner, stronger, and faster than you have ever been. In essence, The Happy Body program will not only make you as youthful as you were at twenty, but twenty as you would have been if you had followed the program at that age.

The same principles that work for athletes also work for ordinary people of all ages.

Philosophy of Eating and Exercising

Steve Dow (54-year-old venture capitalist)

I was looking for a new approach to my health — something that would be easy to incorporate into my life that was not too rigid and not too time consuming. Fortunately, my wife discovered Jerzy and Aniela. It sounded quite interesting, and most importantly, different, so we decided to begin the program together. Actually, "program" is probably a misnomer as it denotes something that you start and finish. I love that The Happy Body is really a philosophy and an approach to eating and exercise that shouldn't ever end. It becomes part of your life. In any event, while I knew I needed to get back into shape, I was shocked when Jerzy told me my body composition. Between that shock, and my wife as a companion, I was quite motivated.

The exercise came easy. Controlling my eating was not easy. Not because the right foods weren't enjoyable or satisfying, but I *love* to eat and I *love* to drink wine. In spite of those urges and following (reasonably well) the eating guidelines, I quickly made good progress on losing fat and building muscle.

Having been an athlete in my past, I realized that what I enjoyed about Jerzy was that he was a coach, not a trainer. This is more than just a semantic difference. I'd never heard a trainer use "meditation," "parasympathetic nervous system," and "weightlifting" in the same sentence. A typical trainer tells you what to do or is there to be your exercise buddy. A coach explains why you do something, so that knowledge becomes a part of you.

After about 9 months, I became interested in going beyond the exercise routine of The Happy Body. Jerzy started me on the long, patient process of developing the strength and skill to undertake Olympic style weightlifting. The body needs lots of time to adapt, a process that can't be rushed without injury. Given Jerzy's knowledge of when to increase my weights, I have not had any injury.

The conventional image of weightlifting is of large, lumbering men. It was quite an epiphany to learn how Olympic lifting is totally different. Olympic lifting is about flexibility, form, and quickness. I love the efficiency of the exercise. It feels like a combination of plyometrics, yoga, and lifting, and you literally work every muscle in your body in one movement. Like The Happy Body exercise routine, I can complete it in 45 minutes. My primary goal is to perform the Olympic "Snatch" with my weight — approximately 100 kg — before my 55th birthday. My second goal is to enjoy as much time as I can with my parasympathetic nervous system.

MEASURING THE HAPPY BODY

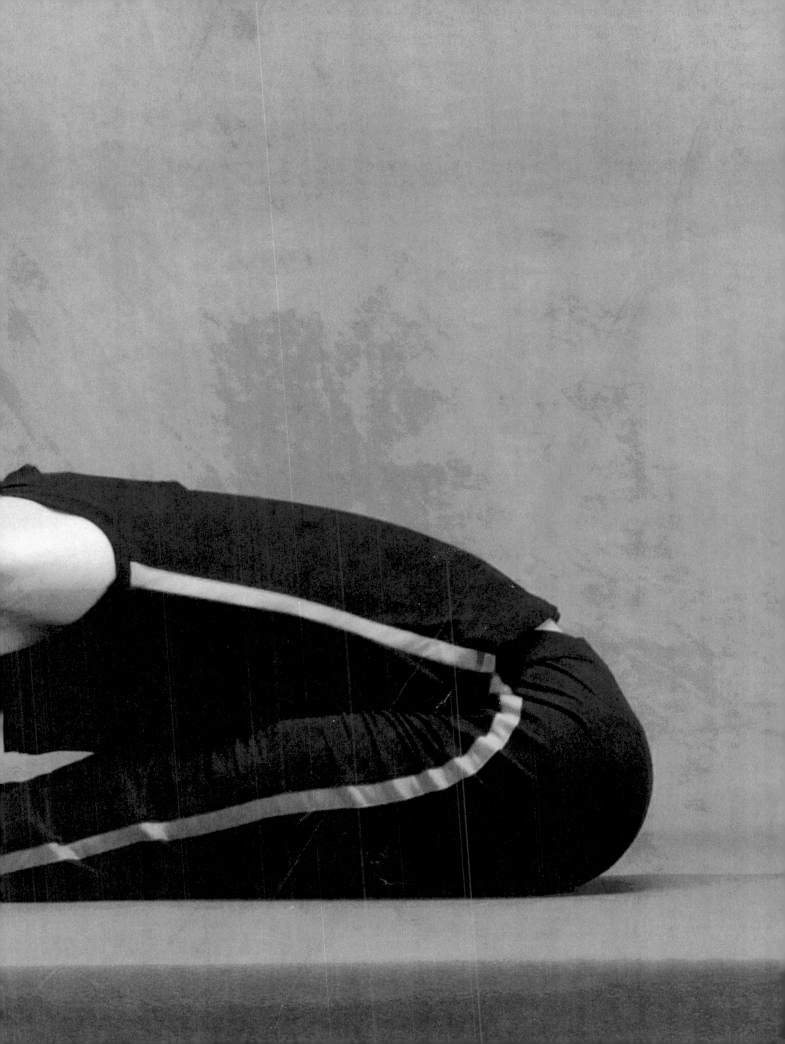

OBJECTIVE STANDARDS

"If you can not measure it, you can not improve it."
– LORD WILLIAM THOMSON KELVIN (inventor of the Kelvin Scale)

An integral step in developing any improvement program is the establishment of objective standards. How does one measure the attributes of youthfulness other than chronological age? We struggled with that question for many years. The answer started to crystallize for us during the 2002 World Weightlifting Games in Melbourne, Australia. After the opening ceremony, and before our own events, we watched the oldest weightlifters compete.

Charlie Henderson, an Australian weightlifter who competed in the 136-pound weight category, was slated to lift 137.5 pounds above his head. When he appeared, everyone applauded. He walked to the platform with his chest held high, his back straight, and his arms loosely at his sides. After bowing to the audience, he approached the bar, lowered himself, cleaned the weight to his chest without effort, and jerked it above his head. We watched with amazement as he held the bar high in the air with straight arms, for Charlie Henderson was 80 years old.

When Jerzy was thirteen, he started lifting weights in his backyard. At the time, he could lift his own weight—122 pounds—something only the strongest teenagers could do. Yet here was an 80-year-old man doing it! The implication of this achievement was momentous. We decided there and then that if we could help our clients lift their own body weight, and retain that capability as they aged—just as Charlie Henderson had done—their lives would be more functional, more healthy, and more joyful. They would be able to lift heavy objects, run fast, and maintain their coordination, and, as a result, they would resist illness and avoid injuries. In short, they would have Happy Bodies.

Recovering from Fibromyalgia

Amy Pietz (31-year-old actress)

I'm a very active person these days. I bike, swim, ski, play tennis, run, dance, and lift weights. Now I live my life without pain. But for about five years, I suffered every single day.

I was your typical actress: skinny from smoking a pack of cigarettes a day, and under a great deal of job stress from choosing one of the most unstable professions in the world. Eating crap when I was unemployed and eating worse crap when I was employed. I was living on an emotional rollercoaster, but I was young and just too busy to worry about it.

It's funny how your body will tell you when it's time to start dealing with reality. I started experiencing chronic pain when I was working on *Caroline in the City*. I was playing the part of a dancer and Broadway actress and had heard that Pilates would help me to look like a toned dancer. I used to dance when I was younger so thought it would be easy for me. I was told that my posture would improve as well. I have a slight swayback and shoulders that roll forward. I started doing pilates once a week, pushing my body very hard for that one day, but not exercising any other day or supplementing with weightlifting or running.

So, for about three years, I stretched all my muscles in my back once a week, causing small tears up and down my spine that became extremely painful. Every time I hurt, my instructor told me to stretch that area, which only damaged my muscles more. Eventually, everything hurt, whether I moved or not—standing, sitting, walking, doing the dishes, paying the bills.

As I watched my 28-year-old body break down, I became more and more depressed. I was constantly being told that it was an emotional problem. I started seeing orthopedic surgeons, physical therapists, hypnotherapists, chiropractors, neuromuscular therapists, nutritionists, acupuncturists, and even "energy specialists." I was lying on ice packs for hours every day, full of anger at spending thousands of dollars on ineffective treatments. I went on powerful anti-inflammatory medications to deaden the pain. The drugs gave me chronic stomach problems. It was all too much to handle. I felt I had tried everything.

When I met Jerzy and Aniela, I was skeptical that simply lifting weights could help me, but things slowly started to change. They warned me that it would not be easy, that the more I followed their directions, the faster I would progress. They were right. I started to have hours, then days, then *weeks* without pain. I focused on building muscles that gave support to the whole structure of my body.

Months passed as I followed the weight routine that Jerzy and Aniela designed for me. I stopped obsessing over cardio workouts and have learned to stick to The Happy Body food program.

A friend asked me recently how my pain was doing. I was surprised by the question. "What pain?" I said. I had forgotten all about it.

FLEXIBILITY

Flexibility is the capacity of the muscles and tendons to elongate or shorten for the purpose of movement—that is, of moving bones in key parts of the body (see Figure 2.1).

However, there can be no movement without strength. We are most flexible when we are infants, but we are also at our weakest at that stage. We have to practice in order to gain the strength to turn over, sit up, crawl, and eventually stand.

We lose flexibility because of how we live, not because we age, as can be seen from the fact that people in their advanced years can be highly flexible and strong.

One time, at a friend's wedding, we saw an older couple dancing the cha-cha. Everyone was watching them because they were so elegant, their movements so smooth, rhythmic, and fast. We were shocked when someone told us that the man was 90 and the woman 93.

After the dance, we went up to the couple to express our admiration for their youthfulness. When Aniela asked them how they managed to stay so flexible and coordinated at their age, the woman said, "I simply stretch and lift weights. Every morning I do exactly the same stretches and lifts. In a way, it's like dancing for me. I've repeated the same movements with the same weights for the last sixty years, so it's easy. The routine has its rhythm, just like music — I love it, and I am never bored."

The man, who had been listening to this conversation, added, "Actually, I found out that it's essential to do the same routine every day. It's easier

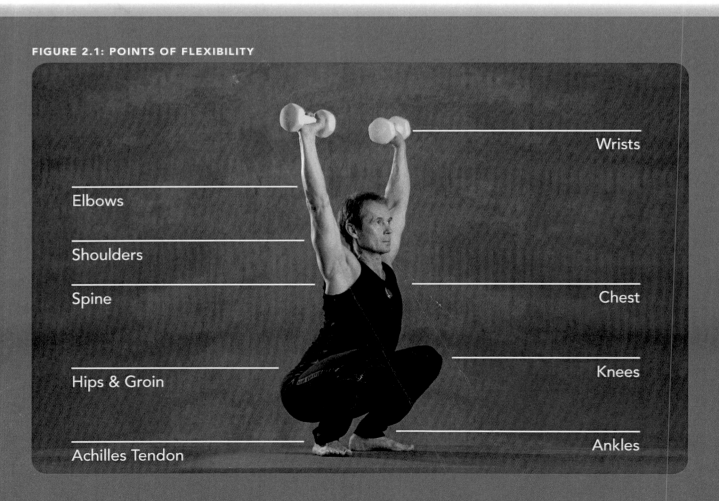

FIGURE 2.1: POINTS OF FLEXIBILITY

Wrists

Elbows

Shoulders

Spine

Chest

Hips & Groin

Knees

Ankles

Achilles Tendon

In The Happy Body program, we recognize three phases of flexibility. First, one has to develop range of motion. Second, one has to develop strength in the movement. Third, one has to develop speed in the movement.

for the body, especially as you get older. Imagine that you learn to play one of the most difficult pieces of music by Chopin. If you learn it when you're in your teens and play it every day, it will be easier to play in your eighties. But if you wait till you're eighty, it'll be almost impossible."

This couple proved that if you do the same exercise routine every day, you will be able to do it well throughout your life. That assumes, of course, that the exercise does not injure you. It must support your body's full range of motion, improve your muscle function gradually, and not exhaust you.

In The Happy Body program, we recognize three phases of flexibility. First, one has to develop range of motion. Second, one has to develop strength in the movement. Third, one has to develop speed in the movement.

A yogi, for example, develops only the first phase of flexibility, aiming more for elasticity than for strength or speed. A power lifter develops the first and second phases, but not the third, by lifting heavy weights slowly. The Olympic weightlifter develops all three phases, lifting heavy weights with speed. Thus, it is possible, like the yogi, to be flexible without having strength or speed. And it is possible, like the power lifter, to be flexible and strong without developing speed. But it is best of all to have developed all three and to be flexible, strong, and fast.

Ironically, to achieve flexibility, strength, and speed, one need only focus on speed, and the other two will result automatically. That is because in order to become faster at any movement, one must increase one's elasticity and one's strength. For this reason, the best ways to achieve flexibility is through movements that involve explosive speed—namely, pulling, squatting, jumping, and throwing. All of these are combined in Olympic weightlifting training.

The Standard of Flexibility

One day, while we were walking on the beach in Santa Monica, Aniela pointed to a toddler stumbling around on shaky legs. Whenever the child was on the verge of falling, she would lower herself into a squat. After balancing her body, she would stand up without difficulty, but then become unsteady again as she attempted to walk.

"Look," Aniela said, pointing to the girl. "She can't walk well, but she has no problem squatting."

We realized that we all squat before we walk, and it is one of the most natural things in our lives, but we gradually lose this ability as our bodies age.

In weightlifting, there are three kinds of squats: the Back Squat, the Front Squat, and the Overhead Squat. In the Back Squat (Figure 2.2), the lifter holds the bar behind the neck, resting it on the shoulders. In the Front Squat (Figure 2.3), the lifter holds the bar in front of the neck, resting it on the shoulders. In the Overhead Squat (Figure 2.4), the lifter holds the bar above the head with straight arms.

Because the Overhead Squat simultaneously improves the mobility of the wrists, elbows,

FIGURE 2.2: THE BACK SQUAT

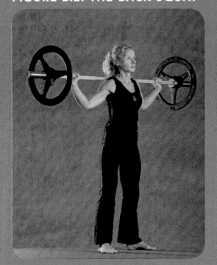
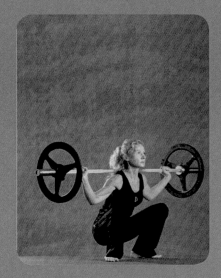
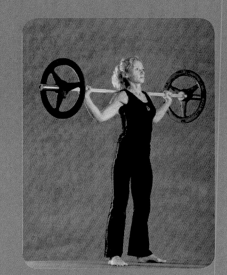

FIGURE 2.3: THE FRONT SQUAT

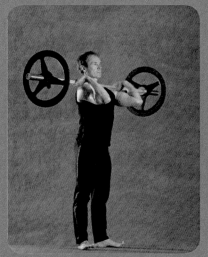
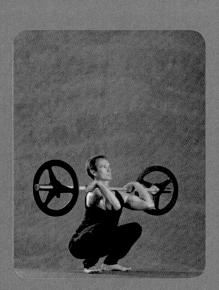
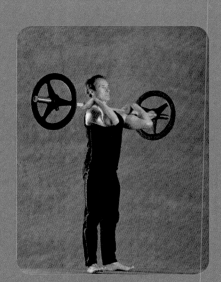

FIGURE 2.4: THE OVERHEAD SQUAT

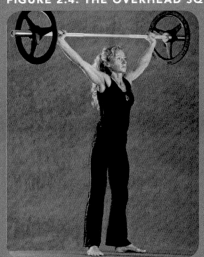
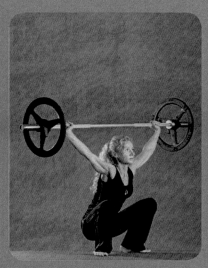
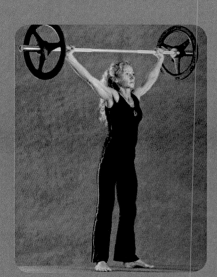

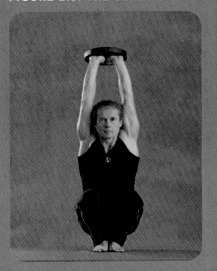
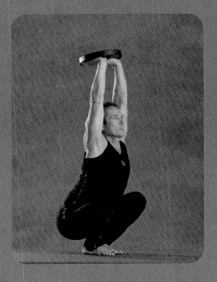
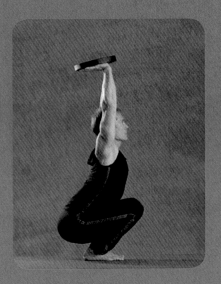

shoulders, spine, hips, knees, and ankles, we thought at first that it would be the ideal test of flexibility. However, while it is an excellent test of strength and speed, it turned out that an even better test of flexibility is a modification of the Overhead Squat that we named the Candle Squat (Figure 2.5), which brings the hands and feet close together, and therefore requires more flexibility.

Degrees of Flexibility

There are five degrees of flexibility:

- Poor
- Fair
- Good
- Very Good
- Excellent

There are five techniques for measuring flexibility:

- The Table:
  Bending forward with an arched back (Figure 2.6)

- The Jackknife:
  Bending forward with a rounded back (Figure 2.7)

- The Bow:
  Bending backward to see the ceiling (Figure 2.8)

- The Corkscrew:
  Twisting the body without moving the feet (Figure 2.9)

- The Jerzy Squat:
  Squatting without leaning forward (Figure 2.10)

We all squat before we walk, and it is one of the most natural things in our lives, but we gradually lose this ability as our bodies age.

The Table

To measure the flexibility of your gluteus maximus, hamstrings, and calves, stand upright with your feet directly below your hips and bend forward with your toes curled up, your knees locked, and your back arched. Then, see how far your fingertips can reach:

- Poor: You cannot reach your knees.
- Fair: You can reach your knees.
- Good: You can reach to mid-shin.
- Very Good: You can reach the floor.
- Excellent: You can place your palms flat on the floor.

FIGURE 2.6: THE TABLE

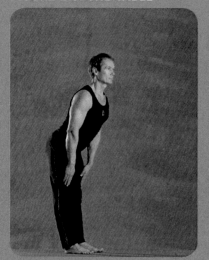

POOR

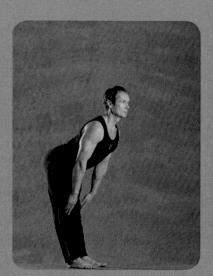

FAIR

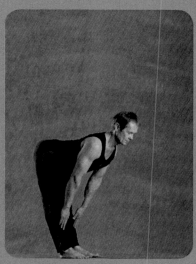

GOOD

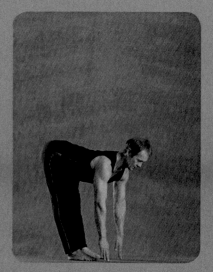

VERY GOOD

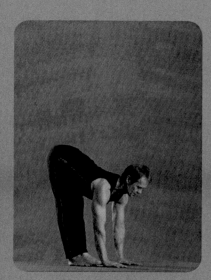

EXCELLENT

The Jackknife

To measure the flexibility of your lumbar spine, gluteus maximus, hamstrings, and calves, sit on the floor with your legs straight in front of you and your toes curled up toward you. Bend forward to see how far your fingertips can reach:

- Poor: You can place your hands directly over your knees.

- Fair: You can touch your toes.

- Good: You can rest your palms on the bottom of your feet.

- Very Good: Your palms can touch the floor in front of your feet.

- Excellent: Your elbows can reach your toes.

FIGURE 2.7: THE JACKKNIFE

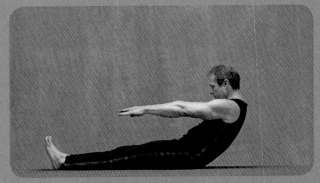

POOR

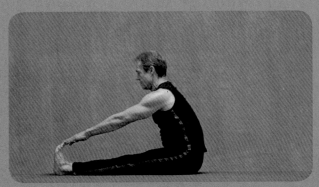

FAIR

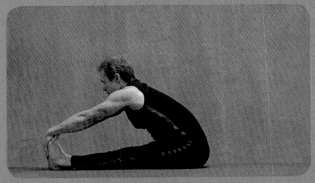

GOOD

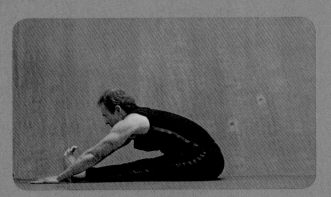

VERY GOOD

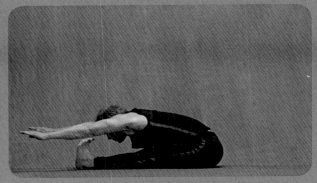

EXCELLENT

The Bow

To measure the flexibility of your cervical, thoracic, and lumbar spine, front of the neck, and rib cage, lie down flat on your stomach, facing a wall, with your palms facing up and your head facing to either side. Arch your spine with your shoulders and arms relaxed, your hands (palms up) and toes touching the floor, and your eyes looking upward:

- Poor: You can look straight down at the floor.
- Fair: You can look at the bottom of the wall.
- Good: You can look at the middle of the wall.
- Very Good: You can look at the edge of the ceiling.
- Excellent: You can look straight up at the ceiling.

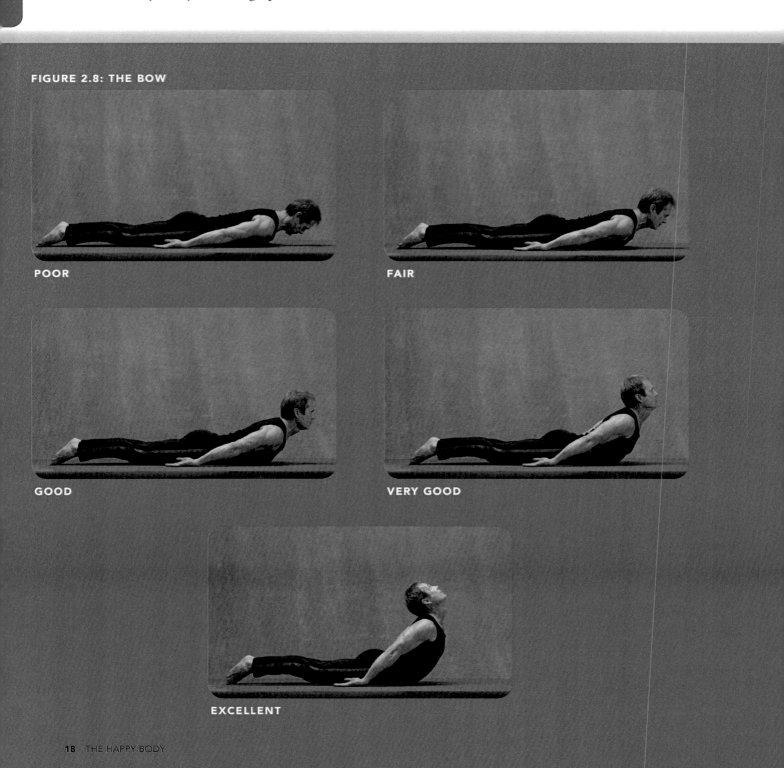

FIGURE 2.8: THE BOW

POOR

FAIR

GOOD

VERY GOOD

EXCELLENT

The Corkscrew

To measure the flexibility of your legs, hips, spine, rib cage, and neck, stand in the middle of a square room, facing a wall. Place your feet directly under your hips, holding a stick behind your neck with your elbows down and your forearms perpendicular to the floor. Twist your body to the right:

- Poor: You can look at the wall to your right (90º turn).

- Fair: You can look at the second corner to your right (135º turn).
- Good: You can look at the wall behind you (180º turn).
- Very Good: You can look at the third corner to your right (225º turn).
- Excellent: You can look at the wall to your left (270º turn).
  Repeat these steps to the left side.

FIGURE 2.9: THE CORKSCREW

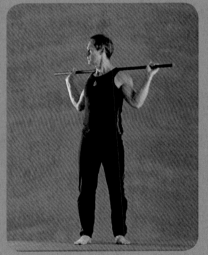

POOR

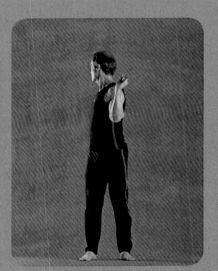

FAIR

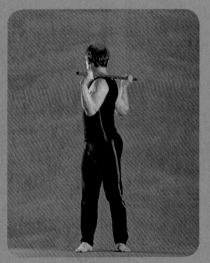

GOOD

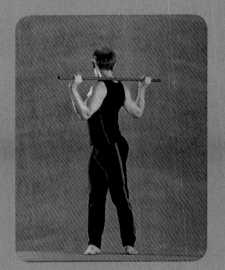

VERY GOOD

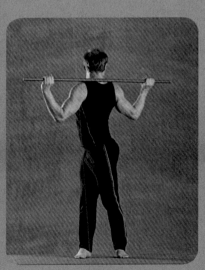

EXCELLENT

Jerzy Squat

To measure the flexibility of most of the joints in your body (fingers, wrists, elbows, shoulders, spine, rib cage, hips, knees, ankles, and toes), stand up straight with your feet together and your toes curled up. Then lift your arms above your head, holding a book on your open palms. Keeping your heels on the ground and your arms vertical with the elbows locked, squat down as far as you can without leaning forward:

- Poor: You can only barely bend your knees.
- Fair: You can squat with your thighs higher than parallel to the ground.
- Good: You can squat with your thighs parallel to the ground.
- Very Good: You can squat with your thighs lower than parallel to the ground.
- Excellent: You can sit on your calves, totally relaxed.

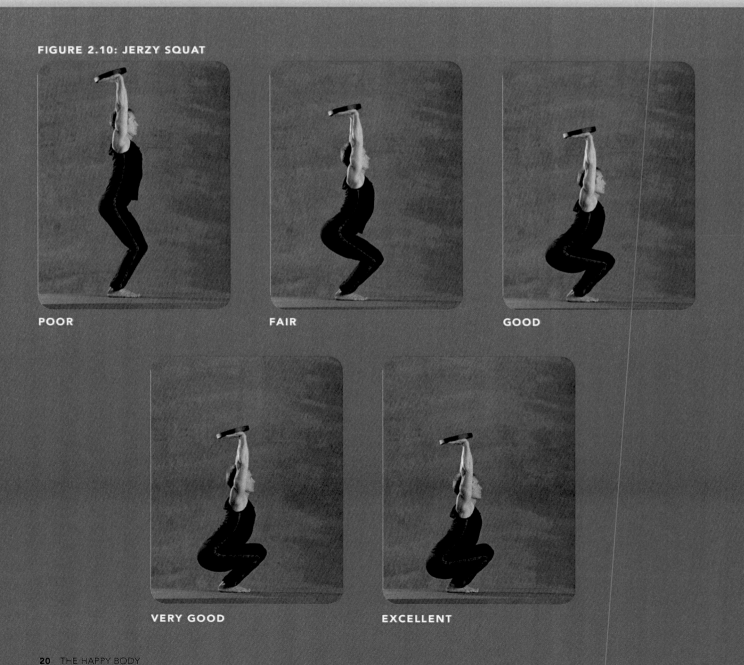

FIGURE 2.10: JERZY SQUAT

POOR

FAIR

GOOD

VERY GOOD

EXCELLENT

Untwisting My Body

Mary Lynn Moran (44-year-old facial plastic surgeon)

My introduction to the enlightened pair, Jerzy and Aniela Gregorek, came about through a friend. After years of struggling with body issues, she was taking back her power and credited Jerzy and Aniela with the amazing and miraculous results. The Gregoreks, she said, were not only skilled at helping people lose weight and become fit, but they also helped with pain and back dysfunction. I had been struggling with back pain that only responded partially to physical therapy and steroid injections. Massage had been the most helpful, but never completely resolved the problem.

The first time I walked into Jerzy and Aniela's lovely home, I thought that I was just going to have a little chat with them about my situation. Instead, I walked out with photos of my twisted body and a "Happy Body Bible" on how I was to live my life from that point forward. They pointed out issues relating to my posture, walking, and lifting that greatly helped me to understand why I was having so much difficulty recovering.

Every week, they would modify my regimen, depending on how my body responded to the routine. I found this feedback incredibly helpful, given the tenuous nature of my back problems. Whenever I performed a long surgery, spent too much time on a plane, or did something to aggravate my back, Jerzy and Aniela adjusted the treatment plan so that I would not only avoid worsening my back, but actually speed up the healing process.

As a bonus, they are lovely people, and I always look forward to my Monday evening meetings with them. Over a cup of tea, we discuss all my recent health problems, and I have a chance to relax with their cat on my lap and their delightful daughter, Natalie, drawing happy faces in my "Bible." I feel so fortunate to have made their acquaintance and hope to continue to share their friendship for a very long time. Meanwhile, all over my little village, I see more and more people walking around happier and healthier, thanks to Jerzy and Aniela's supportive guidance and expertise.

STRENGTH

Strength is the ability of muscles to generate force. Muscles can only exert force after receiving stimuli from the brain. A person who is suddenly paralyzed can still have strong muscles for a brief period but cannot use them because they are disconnected from the brain. Most medical and fitness experts believe that the strength of muscles is proportionate to their size, but that is not true. If it were, two people of the same age, weight, and body type would lift more or less the same number of pounds. In fact, an experienced weightlifter may be able to lift three times as many pounds as a beginner. What makes the experienced lifter stronger is that she has more fast-twitch muscles and a brain that communicates with them faster and with more intensity.

If we were to look inside the bodies of these two weightlifters, we would see that the stronger one has more white, fast-twitch muscle, whereas the weaker one has more red, slow-twitch muscle. Also, because tendons and ligaments are composed of white, fast-twitch tissue, the stronger one has strengthened his joints, while the other one has not.

The difference between these two athletes would be even more pronounced if the stronger one were a weightlifter and the weaker one a bodybuilder. When impact athletes, such as ice hockey or football players, train like bodybuilders, they become slower, weaker, and more susceptible to injuries. When, however, they train like weightlifters, they become faster, stronger, and less susceptible to injuries.

Imagine that you are at an Olympic stadium, watching champion men sprinters. As you look at the Gold Medal winner, you may think, "If I had his body, I could break world records, too." But you would need more than that. Even if you had his body, you would not run as fast, because you also need his brain, which activates his muscle fibers.

When we age, our muscles tend to atrophy and our joints tend to wear away. Eventually, we become weaker and slower, and we develop chronic pains. The only things that can prevent or reverse this degeneration are proper exercise and nutrition, as we saw earlier with Charlie Henderson, the 80-year-old weightlifter who can lift his own weight above his head—something the average 20-year-old male gym member who exercises regularly cannot do.

The Standard of Strength

Although we thought it was reasonable to ask our clients to be as strong as 80-year-old Charlie Henderson, it was not immediately clear to us how to translate an elite weightlifter's ability into layman's terms.

Charlie Henderson had demonstrated his youthfulness in strength by using a move called the Clean and Jerk—a lift that requires considerable skill. Asking ordinary people to learn it would be tantamount to asking them to become Olympic figure skaters. It would also be dangerous. Surely, there had to be another method to measure the strength factor.

Aniela provided the answer. She had been experiencing shoulder pain for several weeks. To find out what was wrong, Jerzy measured her shoulder strength. In a behind-the-neck press, she could lift 50 percent of the weight that she could Clean and Jerk. That was below the 58 percent standard established by Robert Roman, the well-known Russian weightlifting coach. Jerzy started her on a program to strengthen her shoulders. After four months, her pain had faded. By the time she reached 58 percent, it was totally gone. The relationship between the behind-the-neck press and the Clean and Jerk gave us a simple objective for people who want to achieve the first part of the Standard of Strength. Men need to press from behind the neck a weight equal to 58 percent of their body weight. That would be equivalent to being able to Clean and Jerk 100 percent of their body weight, just like Charlie Henderson.

After analyzing Olympic weightlifting data, Jerzy determined that women can lift approximately 77 percent of what men can lift. Therefore, women's goal should be to press behind their neck 45 percent of their body weight (58 x .77 = 45). That would be equivalent to being able to Clean and Jerk 77 percent of their body weight.

Thus, one component of the required level of strength for both men and women to feel and act youthful was established. Most people can achieve it, and once they do, they only need to maintain this standard and not exceed it.

However, our experience taught us that being able to press the required percentage of body weight from behind the neck was not enough for our clients to feel and act youthful. They also needed to be able to perform the Overhead Squat with that amount of weight. But that was still not enough. Even though Aniela could press the weight behind her neck and do overhead squats with it, she still could not snatch it (Figure 2.11).

In order for Aniela to develop more coordination in her lifts, Jerzy asked her to press the bar from behind her neck while in a squatting position and then to stand up (Figure 2.12). This combination of the Overhead Squat and the behind-the-neck press while sitting enabled Aniela to improve the coordination and stability in her hips and shoulders and to snatch the calculated weight.

FIGURE 2.11: ANIELA PERFORMING THE SNATCH AT THE MASTERS WORLD WEIGHTLIFTING CHAMPIONSHIP IN 1999

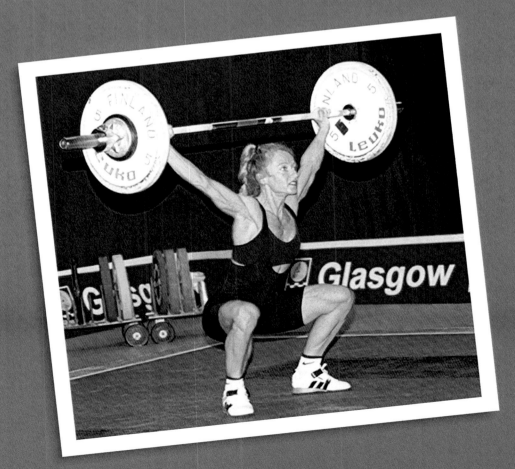

Photo by Jerzy Gregorek

We named the combined exercise the Overhead Squat Press. It is the safest exercise to develop strength because it challenges every inch of the body without requiring skill. It is the gateway exercise to fitness and Olympic weightlifting. In fact, although it is the first and easiest exercise that professional Olympic weightlifters need to do, it is the last and most difficult exercise that ordinary people need to do.

By practicing this exercise, you will not only improve your strength but also your coordination and your flexibility. Indeed, this exercise cannot be performed with strength or flexibility or coordination alone. To achieve it, you must have all three.

The Overhead Squat Press assures that all the joints work together simultaneously and the muscles

FIGURE 2.12: THE OVERHEAD SQUAT PRESS

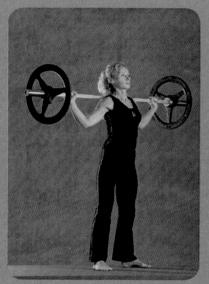

STANDING WITH THE BAR RESTING ON THE SHOULDERS

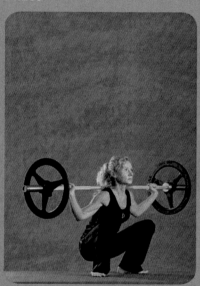

SQUATTING DOWN

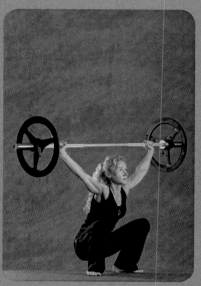

PRESSING THE BAR

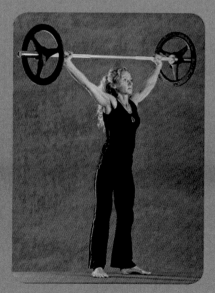

STANDING UP

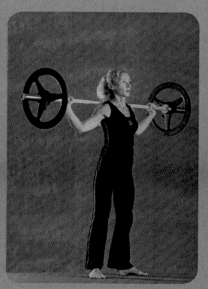

LOWERING THE BAR TO THE SHOULDERS

develop proportionately, improving the posture and preventing postural aging.

The exercise aligns the two parts of the body that are most important for movement—the shoulders and the hips. If either one is weak relative to the other, it will be prone to injury. When these two parts are in alignment, all the other body parts become aligned accordingly in position, strength, and size.

The Overhead Squat Press has become the most valuable exercise in enabling our clients to recover their youthful bodies. Thus, it is our Standard of Strength.

Like every other exercise in The Happy Body program, the Overhead Squat Press can be performed in a minimal space with limited equipment—namely, two dumbbells.

Degrees of Strength

Achievement Level	Percentage of Standard of Strength
Poor:	00%–24%
Fair:	25%–49%
Good:	50%–74%
Very Good:	75%–99%
Excellent	100%

Example: A man who weighs 182 pounds has a Standard of Strength of 106 pounds:

182 x 58% = 105.56 = 106 (53 pounds on each dumbbell)

Therefore, if he can only perform this exercise with 37 pounds, his performance will be fair:

37 ÷ 106 = 34.9% = 35% = Fair

Weight to Lift

Men:	Body Weight x 58%
Women:	Body Weight x 45%

How to Perform the Overhead Squat Press

Perform this exercise in the following sequence (Figure 2.13):

Step 1: Holding dumbbells at your sides, stand with your feet a shoulder length apart and your toes pointed outward. Inhale, flex your abdominal muscles, and curl your toes upward.

Step 2: Without moving your elbows backward, lift the dumbbells parallel to each other until your arms are bent at a right angle.

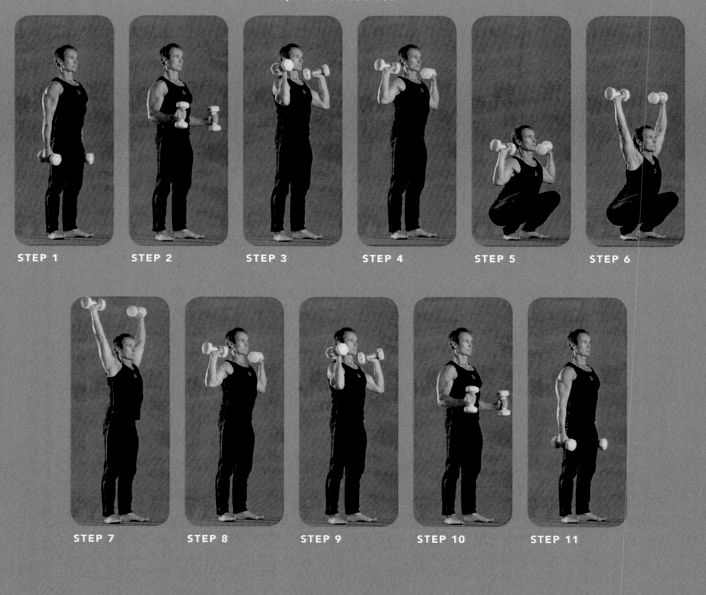

STEP 1 STEP 2 STEP 3 STEP 4 STEP 5 STEP 6

STEP 7 STEP 8 STEP 9 STEP 10 STEP 11

Step 3: Lift the dumbbells parallel to each other until they are at chin level.

Step 4: Rotate your arms backward until the dumbbells are directly above your shoulders.

Step 5: Squat without bending forward or raising your heels.

Step 6: While in the squat position, press the dumbbells above your head until your elbows lock.

Step 7: Stand up straight without leaning forward or raising your heels.

Step 8: Lower the dumbbells to chin level.

Step 9: Rotate your arms forward.

Step 10: Without moving your elbows backward, lower the dumbbells in front of you until your arms are at a right angle.

Step 11: Lower the dumbbells to the starting position, then exhale as you relax your abdominal muscles and uncurl your toes.

Note: When you have mastered this exercise, you will perform it in one continuous motion, without pausing at each step.

Saved My Life in Many Ways

Cheryl Wayne (63-year-old Human Resources VP)

I met Jerzy and Aniela just before my 60th birthday, and I was not very happy about the approaching milestone. I was 40 pounds overweight, working a 60 to 70 hour week, feeling old and tired, and convinced it was over for me. For most of my life I had been athletic; I rode horses and had always felt young for my age, but somehow, somewhere along the way, I had lost my spirit and my health.

The day I walked into the Gregorek's home and met my new coaches, I must admit I was a little tentative. I did not know that day that this was something very different from all the workout programs I had suffered through and all the diets I had been on over the years. None of them had worked. Here I sat looking at these two quiet people; looking at their very simple workout plan, and not realizing this would be a transforming journey for me that would ultimately and literally save my life.

At the beginning of my Happy Body journey, I had my ups and downs and my set backs, but the workout was not hard. In fact I found it addictive because it felt so good. But the workout is just one element of the program, and if it were so easy we would all have happy bodies. The coaching sessions with Aniela and Jerzy were where I met my demons. I had all the well-crafted excuses — I had dragged them with me through the last 10 years and 40 pounds, and I was very good at using them, or so I thought. When I would meet with them, I realized they were not letting me off the hook, and they were not going to abandon me to my resistance.

The physical results from working The Happy Body program were beyond my imagination. I went from a size 14 to a size 10. Emotionally, I learned to thrive. I learned to quiet my mind, focus, and take back my personal power. In fact, one year later I was promoted to the position of Vice President at work.

All of this is wonderful, but as I said before, The Happy Body program literally saved my life. Here's how: A year after I joined the program, I took an extended trip to the French countryside. I was in such good physical shape that I was looking forward to hiking, canoeing, and living it up. I did not look like a 60-year-old — not even close — and I was really excited about this trip.

After two wonderful weeks in France, I was preparing for my return trip home the following day when I became suddenly and violently ill. I had never experienced anything like it in my life, and my husband and I were very scared. We could not leave the next day with our friends, and I was taken to a village doctor. A few days later, I was finally just well enough to travel, so we returned to the U.S. But upon my return, I was still so weak that I went to see my doctor, who ran a few tests to determine what was wrong.

The next day I received an urgent call. The doctor wanted to see me again immediately. She informed me of my test results. I had apparently contracted a deadly case of salmonella poisoning while on vacation. The level of infection in my body was still so alarmingly high she found it hard to understand how I had survived my ordeal. She went on to say that at my age, and with the severity of the poisoning, it was a miracle I had lived through this. According to her, it was only because I was so incredibly healthy and fit, that I survived – an average 60-year-old would have died.

For this and so many healthy reasons, I am forever devoted to the principles of The Happy Body and grateful to Aniela and Jerzy.

SPEED

Speed equals distance divided by time (S=D÷T). To become faster, one must either cover more distance in the same time or the same distance in less time. In sprinting, this is obvious because the distances are relatively long, such as 100 meters. In Olympic weightlifting, this is less obvious because the bar is only thrown perhaps 6 inches up into the air. While it is going upward, the lifter is going downward to catch it. If the lifter catches the bar before it comes down, he is successful. If, however, he is late, he must jump away from the bar and miss the lift.

Over the years of coaching Olympic weightlifting, we have learned that even though some lifters are strong, they still cannot lift heavy weights. The reason for this is they are slow. That is, they have converted their fast-twitch muscles into slow-twitch muscles. Thus, in Olympic weightlifting, the lift must occur within a certain time. Otherwise, it will not happen, or the lifter will be injured. The same thing is true in life. Saving yourself from falling depends on the fast reactions of your brain, nervous system, and muscles. In older people, this brain reaction is delayed by a split second which is enough to increase their incidence of falls.

The Overhead Squat Press, which is the safest exercise for developing speed, will train you to accelerate your reactions and to prevent them from ever slowing down. It will do this by increasing the number of your fast-twitch muscle fibers and the volume of hormones in your brain.

The Standard of Speed

After studying the timing of many lifters as they performed the Overhead Squat Press, we noticed that the average time to perform it is 5 seconds (i.e., from Steps 5 through 7). That became our Standard of Speed. Before you test yourself for speed, however, you *must* first have achieved the Standard of Strength.

Degrees of Speed

Follow the steps for the Overhead Squat Press given above.

Achievement Level	Performance Time	
Poor:	12	seconds or more
Fair:	10–11	seconds
Good:	8–9	seconds
Very Good:	6–7	seconds
Excellent:	5	seconds or less

The Overhead Squat Press, which is the safest exercise for developing speed, will train you to accelerate your reactions and to prevent them from ever slowing down.

Ever Greater Goals

William Stanford (59-year-old businessman)

A year ago I was walking down the hall of my doctor's office on the way to my annual physical. As I stopped at the desk, I heard the doctor behind me ask the receptionist, "Has Bill checked in yet?"

When I turned around, he looked at me with a puzzled expression, and said, "Bill?" "Why, yes," I replied, as it was clear that my doctor of thirty years had not recognized me. Actually, I was not surprised, because for fifteen years he had encouraged me to lose weight, and I never had. So, why should he expect me to appear in his waiting room several clothing sizes smaller?

As his test results would verify, I was also stronger, did better on the treadmill test, had lower blood pressure, and a significantly reduced blood sugar level. Or, as he wrote to me on a note accompanying the test results, "We were astounded and extremely impressed by your 40-pound weight loss and your conditioning program, which you have so successfully followed."

It had taken me a little over six months with Jerzy and Aniela to lose those 40 pounds. During that time, I ate better than I had before and, obviously, from a very different kind of menu. My interest changed from high-caloric, high-sugar, and high-carbohydrate foods to salads, hamburger patties or fish on a bed of vegetables, and a wide variety of other healthy foods. For me, having a snack at midday and in the early evening has considerably helped cut the overall volume of food that I eat which, of course, has contributed to my weight loss.

By The Happy Body standards, my conditioning significantly improved as I progressed from a wobbly squat press with a wooden stick to doing 40 repetitions with a 93-pound barbell. My own yardstick is a little different. In the summer, I am a volunteer fire fighter. Each year, we must pass the U.S. Forestry Service physical test, which requires us to carry a 45-pound pack 3 miles in 45 minutes without running. I doubt if I will ever lead the group, but I am holding my own and reducing my elapsed time with every test thanks to my physical fitness through The Happy Body program.

LEANNESS

Leanness is the optimal percentage of fat to muscle. There are three categories of people who epitomize leanness: athletes, dancers, and bodybuilders. Athletes and dancers become lean to improve their performance. Bodybuilders, on the other hand, become lean to improve their appearance. Essentially, a bodybuilding competition is a beauty pageant. Since life is about doing things, most people prefer to become lean by following the practices of athletes and dancers, rather than those of bodybuilders. Athletes, dancers, and bodybuilders all aim to increase the size of their muscles, but athletes and dancers become strong, fast, and agile by aiming for an optimally efficient muscle size, whereas bodybuilders become weak, slow, and awkward by aiming for ever-bigger muscles, which become increasingly inefficient.

The Standard of Leanness

In Olympic weightlifting competition, it is important to be as lean as possible. As we said earlier, fat does not lift; muscle does. Jerzy competes in the 136-pound weight class. For the eight weeks

that he prepares for the competition, he eats one-third fewer calories every day (1,000 instead of 1,500) so that the other third (500 calories) comes from burning his own body fat. In this way, he loses 1% of his body fat each week—without any loss of muscle size or strength. When he weighs in two hours before the event, as is required in competitions, he has no more than 2 percent body fat.

Does he maintain that percentage of body fat in the off-season? Absolutely not. It would be unrealistic to stay at that percentage all year round, and unhealthy, because he would be vulnerable to the flu, colds, and other illnesses. As soon as the competition is over, he starts to regain all that body fat, at the same rate of 1% per week, by eating one-third more calories than usual every day (2,000 instead of 1,500) until he returns to his off-season body weight. At that point, he resumes his normal nutritious diet (1,500 calories per day), treating himself occasionally to a dessert or an alcoholic beverage.

Jerzy feels the most balanced at 10 percent body fat, not the 2 percent at which he competes

Athletes, dancers, and bodybuilders all aim to increase the size of their muscles, but athletes and dancers become strong, fast, and agile by aiming for an optimally efficient muscle size, whereas bodybuilders become weak, slow, and awkward by aiming for ever-bigger muscles, which become increasingly inefficient.

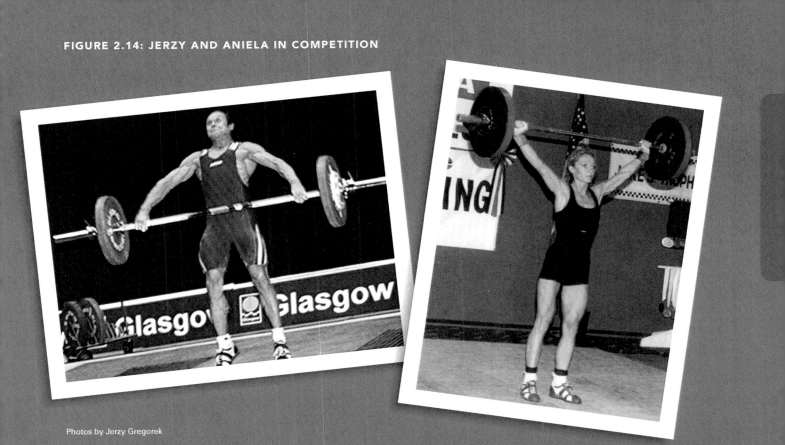

Photos by Jerzy Gregorek

(Figure 2.14, left), and Aniela feels the most balanced at 13 percent body fat, not the 7 percent at which she competes (Figure 2.14, right).

At those higher percentages, we feel relaxed, strong, and happy. Therefore, we decided that 10 percent should be the leanness standard for men, and 13 percent for women, since they naturally carry between 3 and 4 percent more fat than men.

Most of our female clients, from teenagers to seniors, are 35% to 45% fat when they first come to us. Many of them have the preconception that women should be no less than 20% body fat, and they cannot envision themselves below that, even though they have the example of Aniela before their eyes. They assume that Aniela stays like this to compete, and they can never have a figure like hers.

Fifteen years ago, we discovered that many of our female clients would get down to 20% body fat and then go off on their own to maintain that level. However, some months later, they would return with 25% to 30% body fat. We came to realize

that being average, which is 20% body fat, doesn't motivate women to maintain that level. If they achieve excellence, on the other hand, they have something to fight for. The problem was, we didn't know how to persuade them to be excellent.

One day, one of our clients, Mary, arrived at our studio, full of anger and self-righteousness. "You are wrong," she said to Jerzy, "that I should be thirteen percent body fat. I looked it up on the Internet, and it said that I shouldn't be less than twenty percent. I'll show you. Where's your computer?"

Since she was so upset, Jerzy took her to his computer, where she quickly called up the site she had visited at home.

Jerzy looked it over.

"So," she said, looking triumphant. "You see? You were wrong!"

"Alright," Jerzy said, "what do you want to do now?"

"I want to stop at twenty percent."

"And you're satisfied with that?"

"Yes."

Jerzy thought for a moment, and then he said, "Alright, let's look at your progress."

He opened Mary's file on the computer screen, and went to her pictures, which showed her at 41%, 33%, 27%, and 20% body fat over a period of six months (see Figure 2.15).

"You've come a long way," Jerzy said. Then, filling the screen with the 20% image, he asked, "Do you like your body?"

She studied the picture for a good thirty seconds in silence. Then she turned to Jerzy and said softly, "I have to admit I don't."

Three months later, when she was down to 13% body fat, she brought a new bathing suit to the photo session to show off her Happy Body.

Degrees of Leanness

	Male	Female
	Leanness Level	**Percentage of Body Fat**
Poor:	20%+	26%+
Fair:	17%–19%	22%–25%
Good:	14%–16%	18%–21%
Very Good:	11%–13%	14%–17%
Excellent:	10%	13%

FIGURE 2.15: MARY'S LEANNESS, FROM POOR TO EXCELLENT

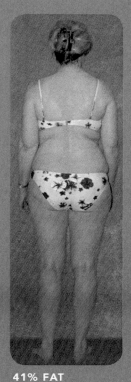 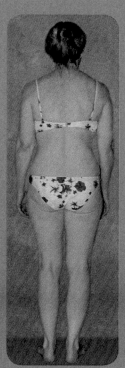 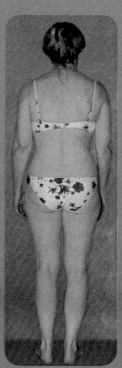 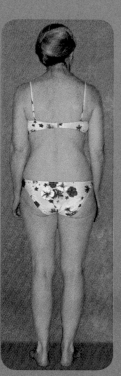 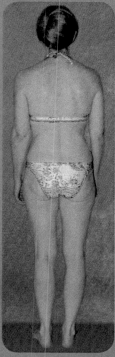

41% FAT   33% FAT   27% FAT   20% FAT   13% FAT

Photos by Jerzy Gregorek

Muffin Top

Sandra Hahamian (43-year-old fitness trainer)

I have always been naturally thin and looked good in my clothes. When I turned 40 I learned that looks could be deceiving. When "low cut" jeans became the rage, I noticed that I always seemed to have a roll hanging over the side. I chalked this up to the cut of the jeans and certainly not body fat. I thought I was making healthy food choices, and I was exercising all the time, but the "roll" just would not go away. I also developed sciatica which was getting worse each year.

When I decided to take the plunge with The Happy Body program I thought I would be in and out the door. I'd lose a few pounds, and the roll would disappear. Was I wrong! Though tall and slim, I was actually carrying around 38% body fat (hello, muffin top...). I could not believe it. I also discovered through the program that I was eating most of the good foods for my body; it was the timing and the combinations that were accumulating fat.

I quickly began to drop my body fat and, combined with The Happy Body exercise program, saw my muscles come alive. My sciatica disappeared. I had suffered with numbness throughout my right leg and low back pain for more years than I can count. Jerzy and Aniela took the time to show me the proper way to perform squats, abdominals, to walk, and to relax. It was simple and refreshing to know that I could make such significant changes in my body in so little time. Six months into the program I was down to 20% body fat and size 4 jeans. No more muffin top!

I have referred many people to Jerzy and Aniela. I tell them all the same thing: You have to be ready to change your body. You cannot assume a quick-fix diet book will do the trick. You have to do the work, respect your body, challenge your old habits, and learn to breathe. The biggest change that occurs during the program is how you think about food. Food is not a soft blanket when you are troubled; it is not a tub of ice cream to soothe your pain. It is fuel for your lifestyle. The Happy Body program creates a whole new way of thinking about food and fitness. It changed my life, and three years later I have not turned back.

IDEAL BODY WEIGHT

Years ago, some of our clients achieved the recommended Standard of Leanness, but still did not like the way they looked, seeing themselves as either too stocky or too bony. The first type would say something like, "I'm lean, but I look like a truck driver." The other kind might say, "I look anorexic." From these experiences, we realized that we had not taken into account in our measurements the relationship between weight and height.

One day, as Aniela was arriving at the house of a client in Santa Monica, a woman approached her and said, "Hi, I'm Jackie. I'm sorry to bother you, but I live next door, and I've never done anything like this before. I've been watching you for months, and I'd like to tell you that I've tried everything to have a body like yours. Are you a dancer?"

"Hi, Jackie, I'm Aniela. No, I'm not a dancer, I'm a weightlifter."

She was surprised, but nevertheless, she said, "I do yoga, Pilates, jogging, lifting weights, and all kinds of diets. I've even had a personal trainer for years. But at five-foot-five and ninety-nine pounds, I still feel fat. I'm tired most of the time, and my body is sore and weak. What am I doing wrong?"

"You feel flabby," Aniela said, "because you have too much fat, and you feel weak because you don't have enough muscle. You're two inches taller than I am, but weigh thirteen pounds less. So, for your height, you are actually too thin. To get the right proportions, you need to lose some fat and gain some muscle, and weigh more than you do now overall."

"I can't believe you're thirteen pounds heavier than I am! How can that be?"

"Because muscle is denser than fat and heavier by volume. So, having more muscle makes you look slimmer. Don't worry about gaining weight overall, because you could be ten pounds heavier and look slimmer."

"Can you help me to do that?"
"I would be delighted."

After that experience, we both had many encounters like that in all kinds of social situations and came to realize that we should calculate ideal weight based on a person's height, using the proportions of Jerzy's body for men and of Aniela's body for women. Once we had that insight, it became easy for us to estimate whether a client should lose or gain muscle or fat and exactly how much of each.

For example, a woman who is 5′3″ tall, weighs 145 pounds, and has 25% body fat would be overweight but not obese. She is carrying 36.25 pounds of fat. The rest of her, 108.75 pounds, is lean mass. According to The Happy Body standard, she should weigh 113 pounds and be 13% body fat (14.69 pounds of fat and 98.31 pounds of lean mass). She should therefore lose 21.56 pounds of fat and lose 10.44 pounds of lean mass.

To take another example, a woman who is 5′3″ tall, weighs 105 pounds, and has 35% body fat would be obese but underweight. She is carrying 36.75 pounds of fat. The rest of her, 68.25 pounds, is lean mass. According to The Happy Body standard, she should weigh 113 pounds and be 13% body fat (14.69 pounds of fat and 98.31 pounds of lean mass). She should therefore lose 22.06 pounds of fat and gain 30.06 pounds of muscle. Although she will gain 8 pounds overall, her body will be much leaner than before and look slender.

The Standard of Ideal Body Weight
The Ideal Happy Body Weights, based on height and gender, appear in Table 2.1. The numbers in the table, which are derived from the proportions of Jerzy's and Aniela's bodies, are based on observations of our clients. Notice that women's weight increases by three pounds per inch, and men's weight increases by five pounds per inch.

Body Height	Female Body Weight (pounds)	Male Body Weight (pounds)
TABLE 2.1: THE HAPPY BODY IDEAL BODY WEIGHT INDEX		
4′10″	98	110
4′11″	101	115
5′0″	104	120
5′1″	107	125
5′2″	110	130
5′3″	113	135
5′4″	116	140
5′5″	119	145
5′6″	122	150
5′7″	125	155
5′8″	128	160
5′9″	131	165
5′10″	134	170
5′11″	137	175
6′0″	140	180
6′1″	143	185
6′2″	146	190
6′3″	149	195
6′4″	152	200

Degrees of Ideal Body Weight

A few of our clients prefer to be slightly lighter or heavier than these ideals, due to bone structure or just personal taste. For them we recommend going one step above or below on the height chart. For example, a woman who is 5′3″ might prefer to weigh 110 or 116 rather than 113 pounds, and a man who is 5′11″ might prefer to weigh 170 or 180 rather than 175 pounds.

Achievement Level	Number of Steps Below or Above Ideal Body Weight
Poor	5
Fair	4
Good	3
Very Good	2
Excellent	0–1

We do not advise going beyond one step in either direction, since a person who weighs too little has insufficient muscle mass and is more vulnerable to illness, and a person who weighs too much puts excessive stress on the heart.

Thirteen Possible Body Types

Very few people have Ideal Body Weight, and of those, even fewer have Ideal Body Weight Proportions. That is, a person can have the Ideal Body Weight for his or her height, but too much fat and not enough muscle, or too little fat and too much muscle. There are very few people who have ideal body weight, ideal body fat, and ideal body muscle, which means they have Happy Bodies. A Happy Body is actually only one of thirteen possible body types. Table 2.2 presents the other twelve possibilities.

It is important to know one's present body type because, as we will see in Part II of this book, to achieve a Happy Body, you must follow the exercise and diet program for your specific type.

A person can have the Ideal Body Weight for his or her height, but too much fat and not enough muscle, or too little fat and too much muscle.

	TABLE 2.2: THIRTEEN POSSIBLE BODY TYPES			
Type Number	Body Description	Body Weight	Fat Content	Muscle Content
Ideal Body Weight				
1	The Happy Body (lean & powerful)	ideal	ideal	ideal
2	The Gymnast (sinewy & powerful)	ideal	too little	too much
3	The Scale Watcher (flabby & weak)	ideal	too much	too little
Overweight				
4	The Lineman (lean & strong)	too much	ideal	too much
5	The Gym Member (flabby & strong)	too much	too much	ideal
6	The Sumo Wrestler (flabby & strong)	too much	too much	too much
7	The Sitter (fat & weak)	too much	too much	too little
8	The Bodybuilder (sinewy & strong)	too much	too little	too much
Underweight				
9	The Fashion Model (lean & weak)	too little	ideal	too little
10	The Twig (sinewy & weak)	too little	too little	too little
11	The Dieter (flabby & weak)	too little	too much	too little
12	The Dancer (lean & strong)	too little	too little	ideal
13	The Mountain Climber (sinewy & powerful)	too little	too little	too much

Finding the Hourglass

Andrea Campbell (29-year-old people operations)

A t the age of 23, I decided I didn't like my body. I was too chubby and shaped like an apple. For 10 months, I worked furiously at the gym with endless cardio and Pilates. I managed to take off 28 pounds and while I reduced some weight off of my arms and around my middle, I never quite got to the shape I really wanted.

After keeping the weight off for 5 years, I got engaged. Having still never quite been at the point where I loved how I looked or felt, I was motivated to lose those last few pounds and build a better body. Working long hours at a stressful job, I could barely stand the thought of adding the 2 hours of cardio per day that it took to get the weight off initially.

That's when my friend told me about The Happy Body. She said that it was a holistic program that was defined by 30 minutes of weights, a balanced eating program, and relaxation. The point was to build a happy body, not tear it apart at the gym.

On the one hand, I didn't know if it could work. I was afraid of getting too bulky from weights, and I was intimidated by the thought of a diet plan. On the other hand, I was desperate for something that would work and fascinated by the various testimonials. The day that I met Jerzy and Aniela changed my life. Through sticking with the plan, I lost the weight, became stronger and leaner than ever, and I lost that achy feeling from too much running. My favorite part is that for the first time, I have an hourglass figure! I finally have a waist and taut abs. On the occasions that I attend a cardio class or ab class with friends, I find that I am stronger and more in shape than I have ever been. I was never able to make it through an ab class before I tried The Happy Body, but now I sail right through.

I feel liberated that I have the key to health, and it's not tied to hours on an aerobic machine. I can come home, and in the privacy of my own living room, do my weights, enjoy TV, listen to music, or talk to my fiancé. When I finish the weights I know the next few minutes of relaxation are purely my time to enjoy.

GOOD POSTURE

Good posture is one of the most essential factors in life. When our bodies are perfectly aligned, we move with ease and are free of pain. As soon as we lose perfect alignment, all of this changes—tension appears, movement becomes awkward, and pain sets in.

Since we are born without posture, we must develop it, then maintain it. The problem is that first because of gravity, it is easier to develop and maintain poor posture than good posture. That is, there is a natural tendency for the body to collapse. Furthermore, unless you enter a profession that requires good posture such as dancing, modeling, or sports, no one ever teaches it to you.

Your posture is the result of what you do. If you do the right exercises, you will have good posture. If you do the wrong exercises—or no exercises—you will have poor posture. Wild animals, on the other hand, because of their need to survive, have been doing the same "exercises," differing from species to species, for millions of years. This has kept their posture perfect—at least until they become injured, diseased, or old. When we ceased being hunter-gatherers and became farmers, we accumulated enough food so that some individuals could spend time thinking about matters other than survival. This led to specialization of labor, and that in turn led people to develop different kinds of posture. Labor that required prolonged sitting did the worst damage to people's posture, and the modern assembly line, with its repetitious motions, didn't help either.

In addition to bones, muscles, tendons, and ligaments, the body has cartilage at joints, as well as discs between vertebrae, which act as cushions to prevent friction between bones. Without proper exercise, your muscles become weaker, smaller, and misshapen. Then they carry less and less of your body weight, transferring this function to your cartilage and discs, making them compress. That explains why we get shorter as we age: the space between our bones gets smaller. Without muscle support, the cartilage eventually wears out and the discs begin to bulge. Then nerves are pinched or compressed, creating pain, cramps, stiffness, and fatigue.

Because the head rests on the cervical discs, the shoulders and arms rest on the thoracic discs, and the whole upper body rests on the lumbar discs, these areas are affected the most by the body's weight. This explains why so many people suffer from neck and back pains. The increased pressure between vertebrae causes many undesirable conditions, including lordosis, scoliosis, and inflammation.

Because the head rests on the cervical discs, the shoulders and arms rest on the thoracic discs, and the whole upper body rests on the lumbar discs, these areas are affected the most by the body's weight. This explains why so many people suffer from neck and back pains. The increased pressure between vertebrae causes many undesirable conditions, including lordosis, scoliosis, and inflammation that can lead to carpal tunnel syndrome, tendonitis, rheumatoid arthritis, and other problems. Structural aging, like any other condition, including osteoporosis, high blood pressure, and obesity, is preventable and should not limit your quality of life. All these conditions can be prevented or reversed with proper exercise and nutrition and without medical or surgical intervention.

What is the first sign that one is losing good posture? Loss of height (Figure 2.16). As the spine and the rib cage compress, the body shifts its center

FIGURE 2.16: STAGES OF AGING PROCESS

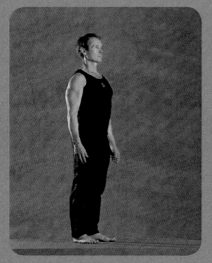

A: GOOD POSTURE

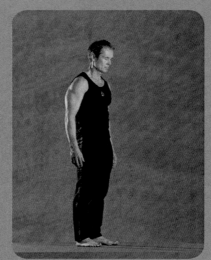

B: SLIGHT HUNCH

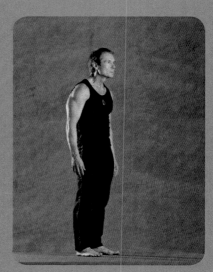

C: HUNCHED POSTURE

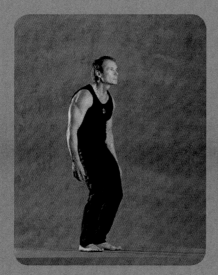

D: HUNCH WITH BENDED KNEES

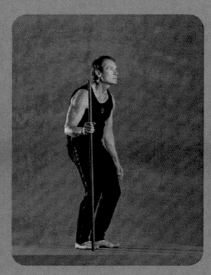

E: BODY SUPPORTED BY KNEES

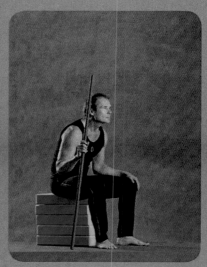

F: WEAKENED ARMS AND KNEES

of gravity forward and loses its upright posture (Figure 2.16b). This leads to the typical hunched posture of old people, but we also see it more and more today with young people, who spend countless hours sitting in front of computers and TV sets.

As we give in to gravity over the years, we bend more and more forward, putting more and more pressure on our lumbar and cervical spines. It is only a matter of time before we have a permanently hunched-over spine that can no longer bend backwards. In compensation, the head, which is now facing down, lifts up, thereby compressing the back of the neck and stretching the front of it (Figure 2.16c).

All of this moves the body's center of gravity forward, shifting the weight from the heels to the toes, which causes instability. This degenerative process continues until the person can no longer see ahead. The only solution is to bend at the knees in order to raise the angle of the eyes (Figure 2.16d).

Now the whole body is being supported by the knees. Since the knees are weaker than the hips, one eventually needs support from a cane or a walker as the knee joints give out (Figure 2.16e).

When one can no longer stand at all because the knees and arms are too weak, one can only sit in a wheelchair (Figure 2.16f).

The final stage of degeneration comes when one can no longer even sit up and must lie down.

When clients first come to us, we take a photograph of them from the side to record their beginning posture. Then, every six weeks, we take a new picture to study their progress. What we have noticed is that, at the beginning, almost everyone is tipping forward on their toes. When we draw a vertical line up from the center of the ankle to the top of the head, the ear is several inches in front of the line (Figure 2.17). In the worst cases, the whole head is in front of that line. Over time, as the individual becomes more upright, the line moves gradually toward the center of the ear.

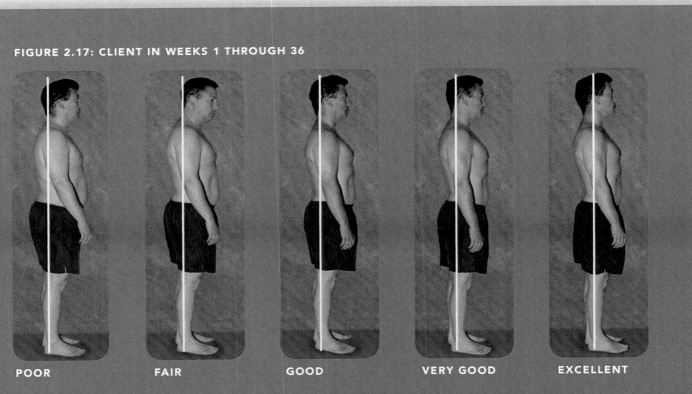

FIGURE 2.17: CLIENT IN WEEKS 1 THROUGH 36

| POOR | FAIR | GOOD | VERY GOOD | EXCELLENT |

Structural aging, like any other condition, including osteoporosis, high blood pressure, and obesity, is preventable and should not limit your quality of life. All these conditions can be prevented or reversed with proper exercise and nutrition and without medical or surgical intervention.

The Standard of Good Posture

When we moved the center line backward, we noticed that people with good posture touched the line at four points: back of heels, buttocks, shoulder blades, and back of head. People with the worst posture, on the other hand, touch at only one point: the buttocks. From this, we got the idea to establish a Standard of Good Posture based on simply standing against a wall.

Degrees of Good Posture

To measure your posture, stand naturally while backing up against a wall, and raise your arms above your head with your elbows locked (Figure 2.18).

- **Poor:** Only your heels and buttocks touch the wall.
- **Fair:** Only your heels, buttocks, and shoulder blades touch the wall.
- **Good:** Your heels, buttocks, shoulder blades, and back of head touch the wall.

FIGURE 2.18: DEGREES OF GOOD POSTURE

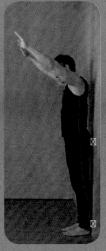 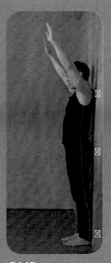 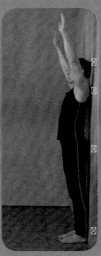 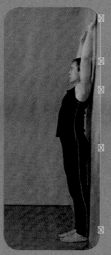 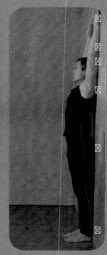

POOR　　　FAIR　　　GOOD　　　VERY GOOD　　　EXCELLENT

- **Very Good:** Your heels, buttocks, shoulder blades, and back of head touch the wall, and your raised arms above your head touch the wall with the back of your hands.

- **Excellent:** Your heels, buttocks, shoulder blades, and back of head touch the wall, and your raised arms above your head touch the wall with the back of your hands and your elbows.

Hygiene for the Spine

For good posture, all weightlifters end their training sessions by decompressing their spines. Normally they do this by hanging upside down, suspended from gravity boots (Figure 2.19). Because this is very difficult and dangerous for the average person, we recommend you use an inversion table (Figure 2.20). To fight the forces of gravity, daily decompression is crucial.

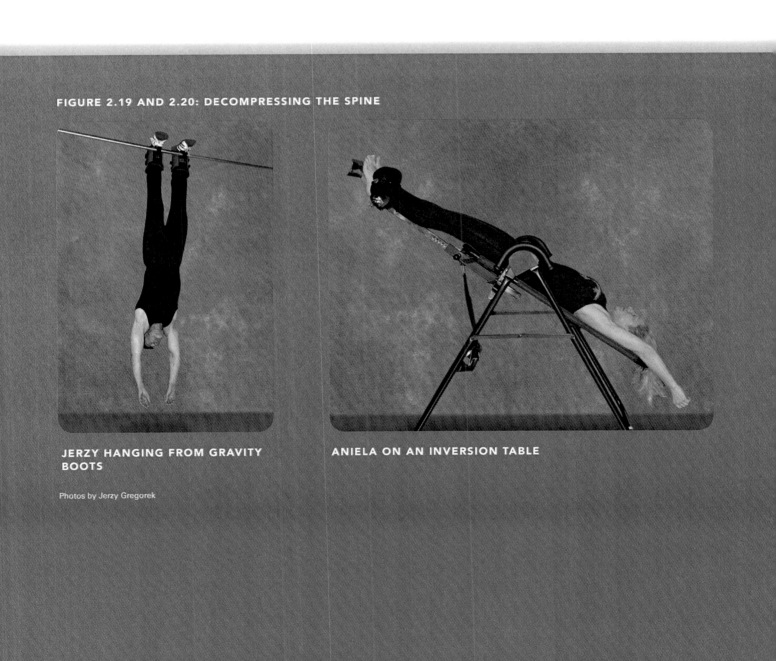

FIGURE 2.19 AND 2.20: DECOMPRESSING THE SPINE

JERZY HANGING FROM GRAVITY BOOTS

ANIELA ON AN INVERSION TABLE

Photos by Jerzy Gregorek

Skinny Jeans

Heidi Roizen (51-year-old CEO, SkinnySongs)

Highs are great in finance, but on the scale, not so much. I spent nearly a decade as a venture capitalist. Through the highs and lows, the dotcom boom and subsequent bust, the only thing that seemed sure to go up was my weight. The years of busy lifestyle, family, travel and stress had packed 40 extra pounds on my body. I was an expert in every diet out there and even did a fair bit of walking, but as soon as I would lose some weight, I'd gain it back — and then some.

One morning I got on the scale and hit a new high. At 190 I weighed more than I had a decade before when I was 9 months pregnant. Cursing myself, I vowed that by my 50th birthday — only months away — I would fit into my skinny jeans again. I knew what I needed was a way to permanently change my life so that I could lose weight and keep it off.

A friend of mine said that one of her other friends had lost sixty pounds on The Happy Body program. I checked out the website and liked what I saw, so I decided to take the plunge.

What I love about Jerzy and Aniela is they help you figure out how to strike a balance between what you love to eat and drink and how you need to tweak it to reach your goals. They were able to help me add some new foods into my life (hemp bread with almond butter—who knew?) and get rid of the high-calorie, low-benefit foods. The things I love, like chocolate and wine, they showed me how to incorporate smaller amounts and still stick to my plan.

Jerzy and Aniela are like high priests of the power of muscle. They are gorgeous living testaments to what weight training can do to a physique. What I love about their exercise routine is that it addresses all the major muscle groups as well as incorporating flexibility and posture-enhancing movements too. And, it can be done at home or on the road with very little investment in equipment.

So far, I've stayed within about a five-pound range since I reached my Happy Body goal. As for my stats: I'm down 40 pounds of fat and up 10 pounds of muscle; I went from a size 14 to a size 8. I've learned to enjoy strength training — I do their exercise routine almost daily and find that by doing so I can maintain the strength and flexibility benefits, as well. I don't think much anymore about "diets." I've found a way to live that keeps me happy *and* keeps my body in a good place.

[CONTINUED ON NEXT PAGE]

While I went into this to lose weight, there were many unanticipated benefits, too. For example, after being on the program and exercising this way for a year, not only did I no longer have any knee or elbow issues, which had been plaguing me for years, but I also "recovered" a half inch of height — I'm now 5'7" again! I just had a body scan a few weeks ago and the doctor told me that out of a hundred of his female patients my age, I'd be #1 in lean muscle mass. Boy, did that make me feel good. Thank you, Jerzy and Aniela!

CHAPTER 3

THE WISDOM OF LOSING WEIGHT

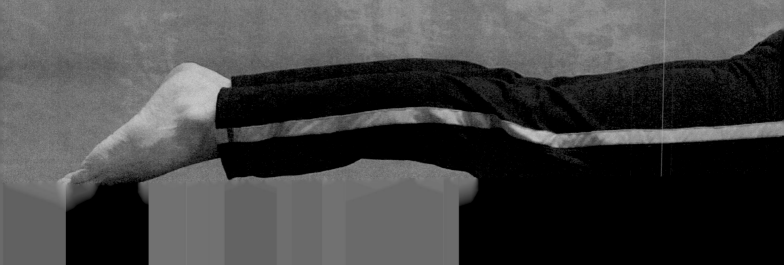

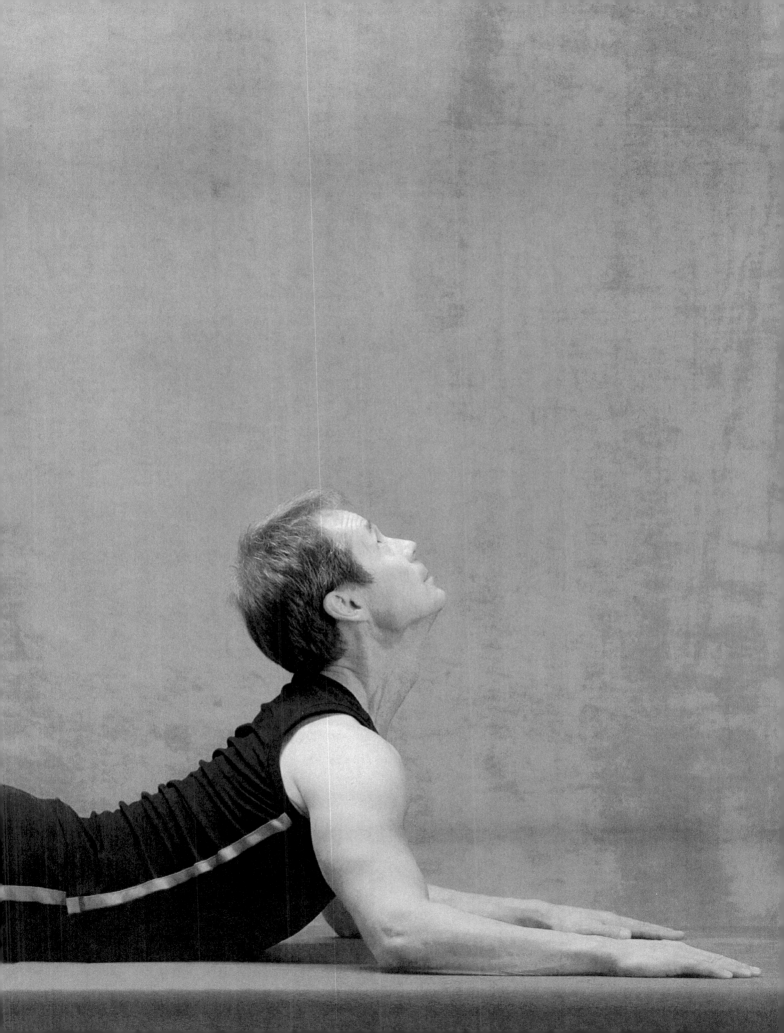

WHEN IS ENOUGH ENOUGH?

"One should eat to live, not live to eat."
— CICERO

Eating properly is a 24-hour-a-day business because losing or maintaining weight is actually harder than overcoming alcoholism. Once alcoholics take that first drink, they are lost — but they can refrain from taking that drink in the first place. With food addicts, however, there is no option to give up eating. To overcome food addiction, one must learn to limit, not stop, one's consumption. Your metabolic rate dictates how much food you need in order to maintain, lose, or gain weight. If you eat a single excess apple a day you will gain fifteen pounds of fat in a year.

Most people have trigger foods, which they cannot resist, not only because of taste, but also because of emotional and cultural conditioning. Germans cannot resist their sausages. Italians cannot resist pasta. Mexicans cannot resist deep-fried carnitas. At one time, Jerzy could not resist piroshkes, which he associated with his beloved mother. Whenever he visited Poland, she would have them waiting, hot and steaming on the table when he walked in. Jerzy would put away plate after plate until his stomach bloated. Then he would conceal his cramps and shortness of breath as his mama stood by, happy and proud.

Trigger foods include french fries, potato chips, nuts, donuts, cookies, candies, fruits, and hundreds of others that you may associate with pleasure. Whatever your food triggers are, you must avoid them totally, like an alcoholic. How you motivate yourself to do this varies from one person to another. Whatever your motivation, it has to be stronger than the temptations of your trigger foods. Otherwise, you will never succeed at losing weight. To lose weight, you must change your whole lifestyle.

The first step is to identify what is most important to you in life. When we asked our clients this question, everyone had a different answer. A divorcee said she wanted to be attractive. A professor was scared because his doctor told him that if he didn't lose weight, he would become diabetic and possibly lose one or both of his legs. A real estate agent wanted more energy to conduct his business. A young mother wanted to be a good role model for her daughter. A student wanted to make his life simpler and more peaceful. Whatever your motivation, you must focus on it twenty-four hours a day.

The second step is to choose something that constantly reminds you of that motivation. It could be an image or symbol that has special meaning to you. For example, you could wear a necklace, bracelet, or ring that is always visible to remind you to do the right things and avoid the wrong things.

But how do you know what is right and what is wrong? The fact is that there are ways to lose weight and ways not to lose weight, and you need to understand them before you can be successful.

HOW NOT TO LOSE WEIGHT

Why is it so difficult for you to lose weight and keep it off? There are several possible reasons:

1. If you lose weight only by dieting (that is, without exercising), you will lose muscle, which will make you weaker. Eventually, you must eat to recover your strength, and then you will regain the weight you lost, if not more. However, the weight you regain will be fat, not muscle, which you can never rebuild without exercising.

2. If you lose weight only by strength training, your muscles will become sore and inflamed, which will exhaust you. Eventually, you must stop exercising to heal yourself, and then you will regain the weight—again, with fat, not muscle.

3. If you lose weight by dieting and endurance training, you will reduce your muscle size and convert fast-twitch muscle to slow-twitch muscle, which will decrease your metabolic rate. Eventually, you will become weak and have to increase your food intake to recover your strength, and then you will regain the weight as fat. Worse yet, you will wear out your joints from the exercise and become inflexible, which may lead to chronic pain that forces you to stop exercising.

4. If you lose weight by being anxious all the time, you never switch from the sympathetic nervous system, which burns lean body mass as energy, to the parasympathetic nervous system, which burns fat as energy. That will cause loss of muscle mass and a reduced metabolic rate. Furthermore, because your sleep will be restless, you will not recover your energy at night. Eventually, you will become exhausted, stop exercising and dieting, and regain the weight as fat. That can lead to chronic fatigue.

5. If you lose weight by chemical means—such as diet pills, herbs, teas, or shakes, which artificially stimulate your metabolic rate or suppress your appetite—the effects won't last forever and in the long run, do more harm than good. Eventually you will have to discontinue using these chemicals to avoid undesirable side effects such as high blood pressure and heart attacks, and then you will regain the weight as fat.

6. If you lose weight by dehydrating your body such as in a spa with heat or body wraps, the loss of weight will only be temporary because the body will demand to be rehydrated, and then you will regain the weight as water.

7. If you lose weight by surgical means such as liposuction or stomach stapling without also changing your diet and lifestyle, you will eventually regain the weight as fat.

HOW TO LOSE WEIGHT

One of our clients, Jack, came to us to lose 25 pounds. After we tested his body, which weighed 173 pounds, we calculated that 116 pounds of that, or 67%, was lean mass, and 57 pounds, or 33%, was fat. According to the Ideal Body Weight chart of The Happy Body program (Table 2.1, page 35), which shows the healthy relationship between height and weight, Jack should, at 5′6″, have weighed 150 pounds, of which 135 pounds, or 90%, should have been muscle, and 15 pounds, or 10%,

The person who is more efficient is also more powerful, has a higher metabolic rate, burns more calories, and handles any physical task more easily.

should have been fat. That meant that he should lose 42 pounds of fat and gain 19 pounds of muscle with a net loss of 23 pounds.

After we told him that, Jack looked at us with disbelief.

"I lift weights six days a week for half an hour," he said, "run for one hour, and work on the Stairmaster for another hour. How can it be that I lost so much muscle and gained so much fat? That doesn't make any sense."

"Actually, it makes perfect sense," said Jerzy. "Working out with weights for half an hour builds your muscle, but then your endurance training for two hours burns up the muscle. During the two hours of endurance training, you not only burn all the muscle that you built with the weights, but also some more that you had before you began training. Therefore, proportionally, you're getting fatter."

"Do you mean," he asked, still incredulous, "that my endurance training was counterproductive— that I shouldn't run?"

"Oh, you can run," Jerzy said, "but you should know that not all kinds of running are good for you. Imagine a sprinter and a marathon runner. Who do you think is more flexible, stronger, faster, and leaner?"

"Well," Jack said after thinking it over, "the sprinter is obviously faster. But the marathon runner must be leaner, more flexible, and stronger because he can run longer."

"Wrong. Actually, running longer shortens the stride, which shortens the muscles and makes them

less flexible. Both runners will be comparably lean, but the sprinter will be stronger because he does more work in a shorter amount of time."

"That makes sense."

"Now answer this question," Jerzy continued. "Do you need to be leaner, more flexible, and stronger? The answer seems to me to be just as obvious. You need flexibility to be pain-free, to perform any movement without restrictions, and to have balance. However, being flexible is not enough. You must also be strong. You need strength to make any move—even to open or close your eyes, breathe, or lift a spoon. Any movement is a combination of flexibility and strength. If you are flexible and weak, like an infant, you will not be able to stand. On the other hand, if you are strong but inflexible, your movement will also be restricted. So, to be fit, you need to be both flexible and strong."

"Okay."

"And there's one more thing. Any movement happens in a certain time frame. The shorter the time of the movement, the more efficient and agile the body is. A person who lifts two hundred pounds in one second is more efficient than someone who lifts five hundred pounds in five seconds, because the ratio for the first lifter is two to one, whereas the ratio for the second is one to one. The person who is more efficient is also more powerful, has a higher metabolic rate, burns more calories, and handles any physical task more easily. While losing body fat, you have to remember that you must increase your metabolic rate. You can only accomplish that by exercising or eating. You could also do it with hormones or steroids, but that would have unhealthy, long-term side effects. Your metabolic rate is directly proportional to the size, strength, and efficiency of your muscles. Only anaerobic exercises that last between six and eight seconds can increase your muscle size and make your muscles strong and efficient."

"Why six to eight seconds?"

"Because our fastest energy comes from a chemical in the muscles called adenosine tri-phosphate, or ATP, all of which is used up in six to eight seconds. You need speed to be agile to react quickly to any changed situation. As you know, aging means losing flexibility, strength, speed, and muscle size, and that adds up to poor posture and a lowering of your metabolic rate. In other words, as you get older, you become stiffer, weaker, slower, fatter, more stooped over, and tired. Running sprints no more than a hundred meters will make your body more flexible, stronger, faster, leaner, upright, and energetic. Anything longer than a hundred meters will do the opposite."

"Alright," Jack said, "I understand all that. But didn't you say that I can also increase my metabolic rate by eating?"

"Yes, you can increase your metabolic rate with food in four ways. First, you can time your meals so that you eat every three hours, but only enough to give you energy for two hours. After that, you should feel slightly hungry. When your body has processed all the food that you ate, it has two choices when it gets hungry. To survive for the additional hour, it can either eat its own muscle, or it can eat its own fat. If you are calm, your body will eat your fat for no more than one hour. If you are anxious, your body will burn its muscle instead. On the other hand, if you do *not* eat after three hours, your body will stop eating fat, as a protection so you don't use all your reserves and die. It's very simple: at that moment, it wants to survive, and so it wants to protect its reserves. Therefore,

if you want to eat up your fat, you must eat every three waking hours."

"How did you come up with that number? Why not two hours or four?"

"We've done experiments with our clients and ourselves, and found that after two hours or after four hours, fat stayed on the body. But after three hours, you can burn off one hundred to two hundred calories. Let's assume you eat five times a day. That will add up to between five hundred and one thousand calories every day. Since there are 3,500 calories in every pound of body fat, that translates into one-eighth to one-quarter of a pound of fat per day, approximately one to two pounds a week or fifty to one hundred pounds in a year! The exact number of calories you burn each time you eat will vary, but the number should be about the same number of calories as your Ideal Body Weight. For instance, if your Ideal Body Weight is 150 pounds, you should burn 150 calories of fat five times a day."

"Wow! Okay, let me figure this out. Hand me your calculator. Alright, 150 times five is 750 calories per day... or 5,250 calories per week. If I divide 5,250 by 3,500, it comes to 1.5 pounds. So I would lose one and a half pounds of fat every week. Since you've calculated that I need to lose 42 pounds of fat, that should take 28 weeks."

"Right. Now, the second way you can increase your metabolic rate with food is to control the volume that you eat. If you eat until you are full, your stomach will expand beyond its normal size. That will slow the process of mixing food inside the stomach, thereby slowing digestion. If your digestion slows, your metabolism slows down with it, making you tired and sleepy. It can be hours before your body breaks down the food and eventually processes it. During that time, your metabolism will be slow, and your body will not burn its own fat. Plus, as soon as the stomach shrinks back to its normal size, it will send a message of hunger to the brain. At that moment, even though you still have food inside your body, you will think you are hungry, and you will begin to eat."

"So, you're advising me to stop eating before I feel full?"

"Right. When you undereat, that prevents your stomach from expanding, which in turn speeds up your digestion and therefore raises your metabolic rate. You will burn more calories and won't receive misleading messages that you're hungry."

"So, that's why I get so hungry the day after I go to a party. I eat too much, my stomach hurts, I have no energy, and I get sleepy. Then, the next morning... in fact, the whole next day... I eat more than usual."

"You got it! Now, the third way you can increase your metabolic rate is to eat *nutritionally complete foods*—that is, foods that contain protein, fat, sugar, fiber, minerals, and vitamins in a healthy ratio. If you eat incomplete foods, some nutrients will be missing. For example, if you only eat carbohydrates, such as fruits, vegetables, or grains, you will lack protein, fat, some vitamins, some minerals, and certain enzymes that are essential for the digestive process. If you only eat protein, you will lack carbohydrates, fiber, and some minerals and vitamins. If you only eat fat, you will lack everything but calories and traces of minerals— no protein, carbohydrates, fiber, or vitamins. To digest food, the body must take the missing components from itself. That depletes the body, slows down your metabolism, and makes you tired. Eating complete foods speeds up the digestive and eliminative processes. Your metabolism increases, and you feel energized and fresh."

"Oh, so that's why, after I eat a bunch of cherries,

I get so sluggish and swollen. First, I get a rush of energy from the sugar. But then, half an hour later, I get tired because I'm not getting any protein and fat."

"Correct. Now, let's discuss the fourth way you can increase your metabolic rate with food. That is to eat *high-quality foods*. If you eat foods that are not produced organically—ones that are full of hormones, antibiotics, and pesticides— the body must first eliminate the poisons, which are unhealthy for your liver and kidneys. Also, nonorganic foods will not have enough vitamins and minerals because those foods are grown too quickly and therefore lack their full complement of nutrients. Again, the missing components must come from the body, which makes it tired and sluggish. If you eat organic food, on the other hand, you will avoid the poisons that age your organs and shorten your life. Organic food supplies the body with enough minerals and vitamins to promote healthy digestion and elimination. That increases your metabolic rate, and you feel energetic and fresh."

"Now I understand why, when I go to Europe, I eat more, I lose weight, and I have more energy. I also move my bowels more often."

"Of course, because Europeans still use far fewer hormones, antibiotics, and pesticides in their food. Not only that, we in America dye, moisturize, and texturize our food; we fill it with artificial flavors and preservatives, and spray it with sulfites, nitrites, and acids before it is made into processed products. We then no longer have produce that is natural, pure and wholesome."

> Organic food supplies the body with enough minerals and vitamins to promote healthy digestion and elimination. That increases your metabolic rate, and you feel energetic and fresh.

"You see, when I come back from Europe and start eating American food, I'm constipated for days, gain back more weight than I had before, and I'm tired all the time."

"Exactly."

"So now, I guess I understand all the principles of The Happy Body program."

Aniela, who had been listening to us for the past few minutes, said, "Actually, there's another point. It's not enough just to eat organic food—it must be *complete* organic food. You could eat organic white bread, but that would still be empty calories. Complete foods are mixtures of proteins, fats, and vegetables or fruits. Complex carbohydrates, such as rice, wheat, and corn are also incomplete and should be complemented with vegetables or fruits."

"By the way," Jerzy said, "complex carbohydrates are exactly what we feed to pigs, which is why they're forty-five percent fat, compared to wild pigs, which are only three percent fat."

"Really?"

"Not only that," Aniela said, "but to digest rice, wheat, and corn without vegetables or fruits, your body must use up its own vitamins, minerals, and enzymes—when you do that, your metabolic rate drops, and you get tired. Then you think that your fatigue is due to hunger, not to missing nutrients. That message misleads you to eat more than you need, and you gain weight."

"But," Jack said, "I was always told that all food is good—that what I need to do is to have variety, but control the amounts."

"Well, as I said, not *all* food is good food," Aniela smiled. "Even if you eat organic food, you still have to have *controlled* variety. Would you like to see how variety really works?"

"Sure."

"What kind of car do you drive?"

"A Lexus."

"Okay. Tomorrow, you'll rent a Chevy Chevette and drive it the whole day. The next day, you'll rent a Toyota pickup truck and drive it the whole day. The third day—"

"Alright, I get it! But food is not cars."

Aniela thought a moment. "Well, then, let's look at it a different way. Can you imagine a sprinter saying, 'Running is boring, I think I'll try boxing'? Or Mozart saying, 'I'm bored with music, I think I'll take up painting'? There would be no Picassos or Emily Dickinsons or Einsteins if people didn't repeat the same things over and over without becoming bored. Perfection is what makes us excellent. As Aristotle said, 'We are what we repeatedly do. Excellence, then, is not an act but a habit.' Whether you're a musician or an engineer or an athlete, you must enjoy repetition for the sake of perfection. If you can master that habit, you will achieve more in life and have more fun."

"You've convinced me!" Jack said. "I want my body to be happy, and you've shown me exactly how to do it. To lose weight, I must train anaerobically and eat the right amounts and kinds of organically grown foods every three hours."

"You've got it!" Aniela said with a big smile. "Now you understand all the principles of The Happy Body program except one."

"There's more?"

"Yes. Relaxation. You actually lose more fat when you're relaxed than when you're tense."

"You're kidding."

"No, there are good scientific reasons for it. Just as everybody knows that they lose fat when they sleep well and wake up rested, the same thing is true during the day. When you are relaxed, your body burns its own fat for energy. If you are tense, your body burns its muscle for energy. So, whether you only want to lose weight and be youthful, or you want to become an Olympic champion, it is wise to be as relaxed as possible."

"I never thought about that. Maybe that's why I've been tired all the time. To have a happy body, I must have a happy mind."

I Can Do This

Barry Johnson (49-year-old interior designer)

It was a combination of things that led me to the fabulous coaching of Aniela and Jerzy.

A couple of years ago, I attended the 50th birthday party of a dear friend. The birthday boy had rediscovered fitness over the last ten years, and many toasts were given to his slim, youthful body. The rest of us had slipped into middle-age spread. That night, thinking about my own 50th birthday which was coming in a couple of years, I realized that I still had time to get myself together. I wanted those compliments at *my* party. Instead, I ended up filing the good intentions away.

Last summer, my family and I took a trip to Portugal and Spain with my friend and his family. I had to admit that I didn't like the way I looked and the way I felt — puffy and sweaty. Meanwhile, Martin had lost his luggage on the flight to Europe and was wearing the clothes of his 22-year-old son. Everyone commented on how terrific he looked.

When the photos came back from the trip, Martin bound them in a book and gave me a copy for my coffee table. I looked like a 48-year-old man who was six months pregnant! Clearly, it was time to take dramatic action. I needed a transformation, but once again I could not overcome my own inertia.

Then one day, I came across an article in a magazine about the creators of The Happy Body program. I liked their strong opinions on fitness and diet. They reminded me of my successful and effective business coach in many ways — goal oriented, no-nonsense — but I still procrastinated, not ready to commit to a strict plan.

Finally, one day at a client meeting, I asked someone about a mutual friend, and she told me that the friend had completely transformed herself physically with the help of The Happy Body program. After many years of being heavy, something in me clicked at that moment. I was finally ready to make big changes.

At my first meeting, Jerzy took photos of me. As with other Happy Body clients, the photos told the truth. I was fifty pounds overweight, big-bellied, and hunched in the shoulders. Jerzy set a time line for me and explained the simple diet. No exceptions; just follow the plan. He allowed me to have the coffee I loved at breakfast and the gin and diet tonic I loved at night. After a lifetime of skipping meals and then grazing all evening, this would be a big change in habits. The first few days felt difficult in some ways, but I was not crazy hungry as I had been before. For dinner

[CONTINUED ON NEXT PAGE]

I would have a great steak and a drink, and I thought, "I can do this!"

The Happy Body plan started with light weights and a new way of breathing during the routine. It felt good compared to the ineffective exercise boot camp I had been doing.

From mid-September through January, I lost approximately two pounds every week. Jerzy and Aniela were so encouraging, pointing out improvements that I didn't see at all.

As I started shrinking in size, my daughter Laura one day busted out, "Dad just wanted all new clothes, that's why he's doing this." She was bothered by my clothes purchases. I was truly trying to hang on to some things, but even my underwear was too loose and had to be replaced — the old stuff was donated or tossed. This was another ritual that helped change my mind-set.

I have found the changing weight routine challenging and encouraging as I have watched my body transform. One of my clients said it well: "You not only lost weight, but your whole body has changed. You are fit." Other friends have told me, "You look years younger." The best comment was, "You look hot!" I had never heard that one before! My doctor was shocked when she read my chart and saw the weight loss, and she was further impressed with the results of my blood work and my lower blood pressure. As a parent, I love to hear my kids now say, "I want to eat something healthy, like dad would eat."

I have now lost forty-five pounds and am toughing out the last five. The Happy Body program gave me the transformation I needed and wanted. My 50th birthday is going to be awesome!

CHAPTER 4

THE WISDOM OF EXERCISE

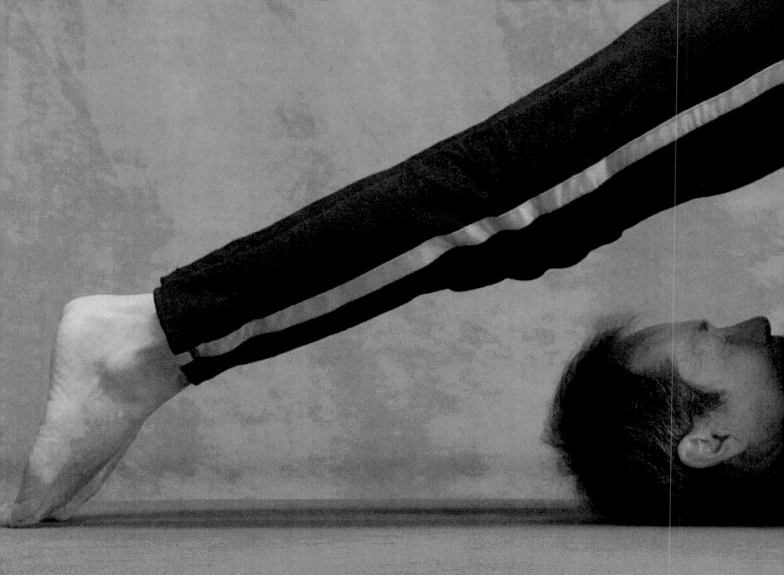

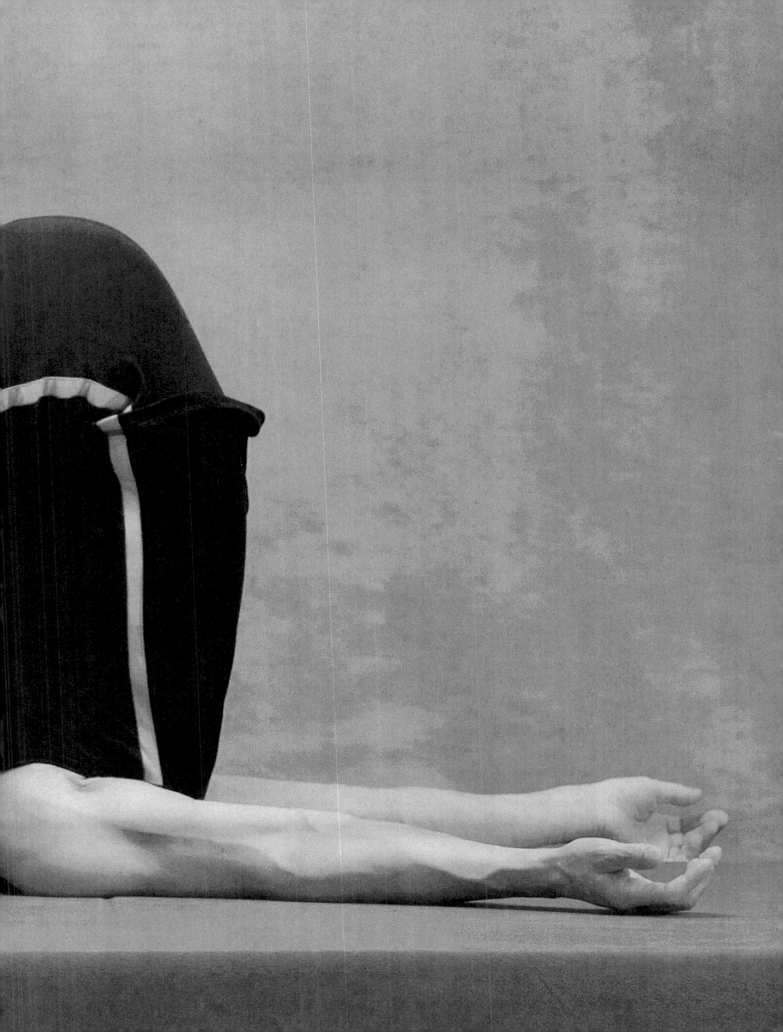

A NEVER-ENDING CYCLE OF FAILURE

"We are what we repeatedly do. Excellence, then, is not an act but a habit."
— ARISTOTLE

Most people think of exercise as a way of burning calories. If they eat too much on the weekend, they figure they can burn it off on Monday. This belief about exercise is a total misconception. First of all, it could take one to two hours just to burn off the calories from one bagel — someone might never catch up with his bad eating habits. The more they eat, the more they exercise, in a never-ending cycle of failure. They cannot succeed in this way any more than they could if they practiced the piano to burn off calories. The fact is that you will never lose weight through exercise. Only after you surrender to this truth can you begin the real work of exercise, which is to make your body as efficient and youthful as possible. Thus, the first step to exercising properly is to give up popular but false beliefs about it and understand its true purpose.

In making our bodies as efficient and youthful as possible, proper exercise helps the body resist the ravages of aging, both mental and physical. What do people think of when they think of aging? We have talked over the years with athletes, health professionals, and clients about this, and almost everyone has pointed to hardening—hardening of the body as we get older: of the skin, the muscles, and the bones. The skin becomes less elastic; the muscles become tight, and the bones become brittle. We are born soft and die hard.

This aging process begins as early as the school years, when children are made to sit quietly at desks for many hours at a time. Many of them round their backs when they sit, which places great stress on their spines and starts to deteriorate their posture. The exceptions to this are those kids who take ballet lessons, horseback riding, or gymnastics. After school, most children continue sitting to do their homework, to play computer games, to play musical instruments, to watch TV, and to eat dinner—a whole day of sitting!

The first signs of aging for most people are mild physical discomforts of some kind. They will say they have a knot in their back, or a stiff neck, or a sore shoulder, or tight hamstrings. Or perhaps they cannot straighten their arms, knees, or elbows. These are all variations of the same phenomenon: some part of the body is hardening.

To seek relief, they get massages to have their tension knots released in their muscles; they get acupuncture to unblock energy channels, or they go to chiropractors to have their joints realigned. When the problems persist or worsen, they may visit a physician to obtain medicines to alleviate their musculoskeletal pains. They may even undergo surgery to have calcium deposits removed, disks repaired, or joints smoothed or replaced. Sometimes these procedures help. But if our lifestyles are out of balance, most of these conditions will become recurrent. Even worse, the hardening can become internal. Our bodies can age in subtle and more dangerous ways, often without pain or obvious symptoms, as in arteriosclerosis and osteoporosis. For these conditions, modern medicine offers hormonal and other drug treatments.

To correct this steady decline, or to prevent it in the first place, people try out all kinds of exercise. The problem is that some forms of exercise make us better, and some make us worse. For example, compare sprinting and marathon running. Sprinters are the fastest of runners and use the widest range of motion in their legs. Marathon runners, at the other extreme, are the slowest of runners and use the narrowest range of motion in their legs. While they are running, sprinters' bodies are as hard as possible during the moment of impact with the ground, and then as soft as possible when they fly through the air between strides. The gap between the hardness and softness of the sprinters' muscles is extreme,

as is the speed with which they go from one to the other. In contrast, marathon runners' bodies are far less hard at impact and far less soft during flight. These principles carry over to when the runners are not racing. At rest, sprinters have the most flexible bodies of all runners and the softest of all muscles, whereas marathon runners have the least flexible bodies and the hardest of all muscles. Similar contrasts could be made between divers and long-distance swimmers, ski jumpers and cross-country skiers, or bicycle sprinters and long-distance road cyclists. Thus, all interval exercises make us better by increasing our youthfulness, and all endurance exercises make us worse by contributing to our hardening and aging process.

The common misconception, among doctors as well as the general public, is that only endurance exercises have cardiovascular benefits. The truth is that both interval and endurance exercises have cardiovascular benefits, but the former has them without the side effects of exhaustion, inflammation, and musculoskeletal degeneration. In fact, interval exercises are better for the heart than endurance exercises because the range between the highest and the lowest number of heartbeats is far greater, and therefore the muscles of the heart are made stronger.

SLOWING DOWN THE AGING PROCESS

The whole purpose of The Happy Body program is to slow down the aging process by retaining the body's softness when it is relaxed while simultaneously developing its hardness for action. The bigger the gap between a body's hardness and softness, the better; and the faster one can go from one to the other, the healthier, more elastic, and more powerful the body. A weak, brittle body is like a solid glass ball. Throw it against a wall and it will shatter. A strong, elastic body is like a rubber ball. Throw it against a wall and it will bounce back with force.

The common misconception among doctors, as well as the general public, is that only endurance exercises have cardiovascular benefits. The truth is that both interval and endurance exercises have cardiovascular benefits, but the former has them without the side effects of exhaustion, inflammation, and musculoskeletal degeneration.

The Happy Body exercises are designed to have multiple purposes, each one geared to one of the Standards of Youthfulness. For example, when people seek to be lean and strong and to attain their Ideal Body Weight, it is important that they lose fat, not muscle. The Happy Body program achieves this by using resistance exercises that strengthen and build the muscles, making it impossible to burn them for energy. Furthermore, every exercise repetition is preceded by inhalation and followed by exhalation, during both of which the body achieves complete relaxation. During these intervals, the body burns fat for its fuel. Endurance programs, on the other hand, cause muscle loss because people continuously exercise without any periods of relaxation.

The Happy Body program promotes flexibility by using exercises that are based on four primary movements: pressing, pulling, squatting, and bending, which we all do in our everyday lives. In order to allow people to increase their flexibility gradually without injuring themselves, every exercise has five levels of difficulty from poor to excellent. At each level, our clients conclude each exercise by attempting to go slightly beyond their current limits, which we call extension. By extending themselves gradually in this way, they progress up the levels of difficulty until they achieve full range of motion in every joint of the body.

The Happy Body program promotes good posture by requiring exercisers to curl up their toes and raise their chests for all lifting exercises. This shifts the weight to the heels, forcing the body into a more upright position. Then, by tightening their abdominal and buttock muscles, Happy Body exercisers align their spines in a neutral position, which eliminates the need for awkward bodily compensations. At the end of the lifts, the exercisers extend themselves slightly further, which increases the body's vertical alignment.

After the exercisers have attained full range of motion in every joint, The Happy Body program promotes speed by having them spend less time on the movement of every repetition and more time on rest and relaxation.

Finally, there is a spiritual component to The Happy Body program, which is essential to slowing down the aging process. As our clients perform the exercises on a daily basis, their lives develop a rhythm in which they start to become calmer, more meditative, more relaxed, and more mindful. Having previously hated exercise, they now look forward to it. Their fitness and well-being are now totally within their own control—and they know it.

Now I Like Myself Better

Tony Abbis (71-year-old marketing consultant)

Through the years, I have always been active in sports — soccer, cricket, tennis, individual skiing, distance running — and had always been in the 170 to 176 pound weight range. With time, a by-pass operation, and a torn knee meniscus, though, I was down to just walking and playing doubles for exercise. I drifted between 186 to 192 pounds. I did not like myself, and my wife and I were looking for a change in lifestyle that would support the energy and activities that we both enjoyed. The diets we had tried were not effective long-term. They did not support our sports activities and induced cravings for "forbidden foods."

For my 70th birthday my wife gave me a three-month session with a personal trainer to see if we could develop an exercise program that would build flexibility and strength and reduce my dimensions. The results: aches, pains, and exhaustion, plus a feeling of futility over the grind of the routines. Lamenting the state of dissatisfaction one day, a friend he told me of his experience with Jerzy and Aniela's Happy Body program. It was 180 degrees different than what I was going through.

We decided to forego a planned visit to a spa and try The Happy Body program instead. The positive impact of the program was immediate. We started to lose weight, we had more energy, and the exercises were interesting and varied. Plus, we exercised at home, and it only took 45 minutes. Within 2 months I was 10 pounds lighter, had gained 6 pounds of muscle, and had a spring in my step again. The quality of my tennis game improved so much I started playing singles again… and winning!

More proof of success is the reduction in medication that I had been taking to control my blood pressure and cholesterol levels. My doctor has currently stopped two of my cholesterol medications and reduced another by half. I have completely stopped needing to take two of the blood pressure medications, reversing my trend over the last few years of taking more and more pills.

I now like myself better, too. The weight loss (without food cravings, I should add) has reduced my belt size by 3 notches, and I feel that I have claimed back 15 years of my life. I am moving steadily towards my target weight and continuing to enjoy the exercises. I feel I am building a solid fitness base so I can enjoy the quality of life that I seek.

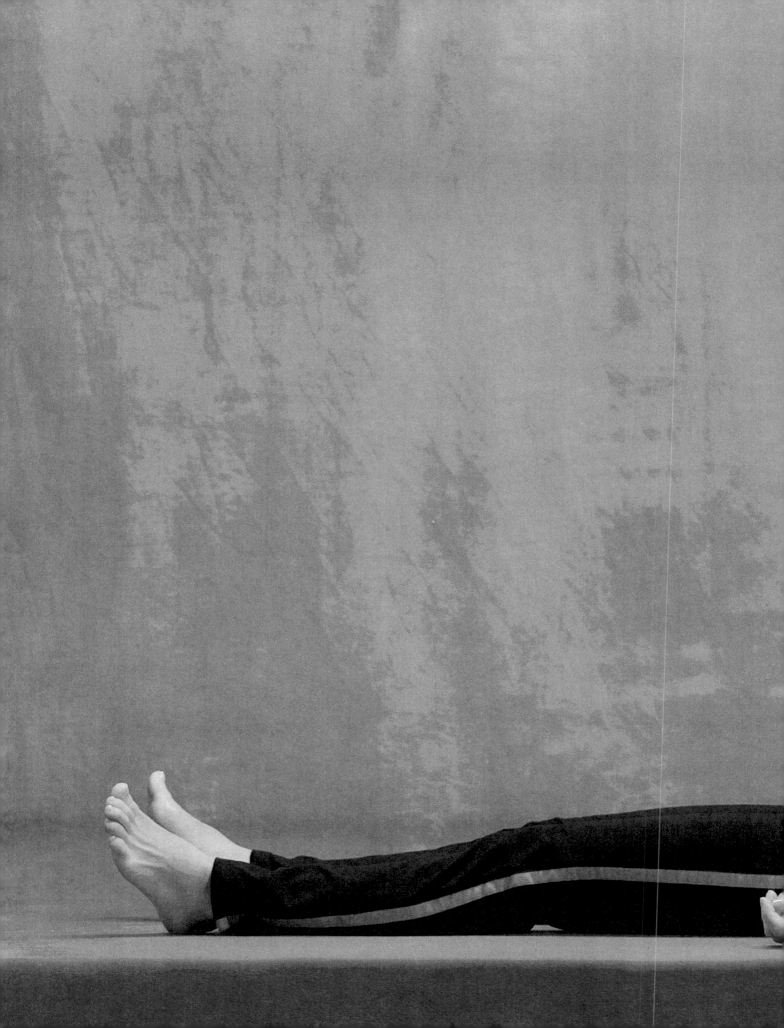

CHAPTER 5

THE WISDOM OF RECOVERY

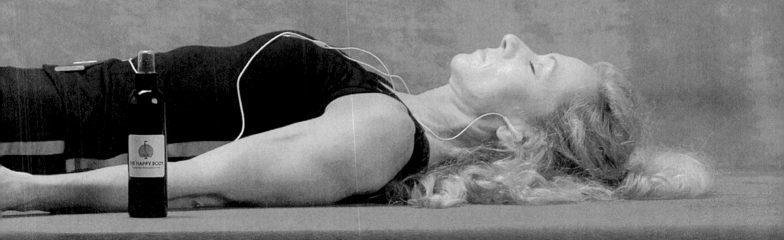

STOPPING AT THE RIGHT POINT

"A field that has rested gives a bountiful crop."
– OVID

The most important factor in improving and maintaining performance of any kind is recovery. This includes both physical and mental improvement and maintenance. Ernest Hemingway said that when he was writing, he would continue until he reached a creative peak, then he would stop. Years of experience taught him when that moment arrived. He knew that he had stopped at the right point when he sat down the next day to write again and found that his writing was effortless. In between, his mind had processed new images and new situations automatically, both when he was awake and when he was asleep and dreaming. Hemingway understood the process of recovery. He would stop writing before burning out so he could face the blank page.

This same principle applies to artists of all kinds, to athletes, and, in fact, to anyone who works. Artists have more difficulty in seeing this than, let's say athletes, because they cannot so easily measure their results. But an athlete such as a sprinter can see precisely how he or she is speeding up or slowing down.

The better the athlete, the more intense the training, and therefore, the shorter the training time. On the other hand, he will need more time to recover because his performance is more intense and so uses up more energy, muscles, hormones, and nutrients. In fact, his whole body, including his brain, will be exhausted at the end of the training session, even though his performance may take only 100 seconds of his 40-minute workout. The rest is rest.

For example, a sprinter whose personal best record is 10 seconds for the 100 meter dash runs more intensely than a runner whose personal best record is 11 seconds. The faster runner will need more time to recover between runs and will perform fewer runs per day. However, if in any particular run, both of them finish the 100 meter dash in 11 seconds, the one who is capable of running faster will require less time to recover, since, unlike the other one, he will not expend 100% of his energy to accomplish the task.

Most athletes are driven to work harder than they should to achieve their goals. Therefore, they burn themselves out or injure themselves and never achieve their goals. Athletic coaches have to adjust on a daily basis the amount of work and recovery their athletes require to improve. The whole point of having a good coach is to have someone who stops you from overworking and sees to it that you get enough recovery.

Like athletes, most people are driven to perform well in their work, whatever it is, but they are unaware of the importance of recovery. They just know that there is something wrong with their way of living. They may be tired all the time, sore, or in pain. When these problems affect their livelihood or their lifestyle, they start to look around for solutions. Most people will start by seeing a doctor, chiropractor, dietician, massage therapist, life coach, or psychotherapist. These people may help them to some degree, but the underlying problem of insufficient recovery still needs to be addressed.

For ordinary people, their jobs are their primary contest. For example, worker A, who uses 100% of her energy to do her job, will go home totally exhausted. Then she will probably overeat, thinking that this will restore her energy, but just the opposite happens. She becomes even more tired, does no exercise, and either passively watches TV or goes to sleep. Over time, she is likely to develop chronic pains, become prone to injuries or illness, develop a food addiction, gain weight, and miss workdays. Her 100% gradually declines to 90%, and then to 80%, and so on, until her life is inefficient drudgery.

On the other hand, worker B, who only uses 60% of her energy to do the same job, will recover as she goes along and will always be fresh. In fact, she will have the option of working harder and thereby earning more money or a promotion, or both. When she goes home, she has energy for exercise, is refreshed by eating, and wants to spend active quality time with her family and friends. Clearly, B is stronger than A, recovers faster and more completely, and has a more rewarding life. Over time, she will become even stronger and then she will be able to perform her job with only 50% of her energy, or perhaps even 40%, and her life will be effortless.

During the part of the day when we are not running or working, we recover in three basic ways: proper exercise, proper nutrition, and relaxation. Proper exercise makes us stronger and more youthful. Proper nutrition replenishes all the nutrients and hormones we have used up. Finally,

If you want to improve your performance of any kind, you must control your rest as well as your work.

meditation, massage, and hot baths help us to relax during the day and to get a good night's sleep.

If you want to improve your performance of any kind, you must control your rest as well as your work. On the other hand, if you rest too much, you will not have done enough work to improve your performance. So to find the right balance between your performance and your recovery, you must observe your accomplishments on a daily, weekly, monthly, and yearly basis, and determine at which points your performance failed to improve. Those failures are the result of either too much work and not enough recovery or too little work and too much recovery.

We see both of these problems when our clients first come to us. Take for example, Michael, a 55-year-old urological surgeon, who came to us complaining of fatigue. He was performing two surgeries a day. Whereas he used to be able to do this without a problem, now he was completely exhausted at the end of the day.

He attributed this decline to aging, however we immediately saw that he had poor posture; was at least 50 pounds overweight; was breathing heavily, and looked intense but tired. He also spoke very quickly—almost nonstop. In talking to him, we discovered that he jogged or swam an hour a day; his diet was full of fat and sugar; his meals were sporadic, and he was not sleeping well. While he was performing surgery, he said, his lower back and shoulders hurt. Since he often had to make life-and-death decisions, he was concerned that his physical problems might ultimately reduce his mental clarity.

The first thing we told him was that he needed to become stronger, because everything he was doing was making him weaker. To begin with, he should stop jogging and swimming, because they were only reducing his muscle mass. He insisted that swimming was his only source of relaxation and asked if there was any way he could keep doing it. We suggested that he mostly swim for pleasure, but that if he really wanted to use it for occasional

exercise, he should alternate swimming every lap with two minutes of rest, and that he do no more than ten laps in a session. Next, we put him on The Happy Body exercise and nutrition program to increase his strength, muscle size, and flexibility, and to improve his posture, and to reduce his weight. Finally, we taught him several relaxation techniques.

After six months, Michael lost 45 pounds of fat, gained 15 pounds of muscle, doubled his strength, became pain-free, slept soundly, and woke up fully refreshed. His posture improved, even when he was performing surgery, so he expended less energy on each operation and could now easily perform two a day again.

Susan, another client, is a part-time college teacher. She works too little and recovers too much. When she first came to us, at the age of 42, our first impression of her was that she was depressed. She told us that she never liked to exercise, and even the idea of exercise was repugnant to her. What she loved to do was go to concerts and museums, read books, meditate, and go to fine restaurants. As her dress size got bigger and bigger, she became weaker, and her life gradually became more passive. She stayed home more and went out less. Worst of all, she was constantly feeling exhausted, which she blamed on her weight.

When we measured her, we found that, at 5′5″ and 129 pounds, 39% (50.3 pounds) was fat and 61% (78.7 pounds) was lean mass. At her height, her Ideal Body Weight should have been 119 pounds with 13% (15.5 pounds) body fat and 87% (103.5 pounds) lean mass. Thus, she needed to lose 34.8 pounds of fat and gain 24.8 pounds of lean mass.

We told her that because she didn't exercise, she was losing muscle mass, and that was the cause of her exhaustion, not the excess pounds of fat. In other words, her lack of strength did not allow her to recover properly even from her minimum expenditure of energy. She was like a big car with

> # The more relaxed we are after we exercise, the more fat we burn.

a small engine. To get stronger, she would need to become more muscular, and for that she would need to do proper exercise.

We explained to Susan that, because it is more difficult to gain muscle mass than to lose fat, it takes more time, and we would have to work with her in two stages. The first stage would be for her to lose 10 pounds overall to bring her down to her Ideal Body Weight. At a weekly loss of 1% of her Ideal Body Weight, that would take her approximately nine weeks (10 ÷ 1.19 = 8.4).

Then, in the second stage, we would work to get her to her Ideal Body Weight Proportions. This second stage would last at least two years, because people can gain, at best, 10% of their Ideal Body Weight in muscle every year. In Susan's case, that would be 12 pounds per year (119 x .1 = 11.9). Once, after nine weeks, she got down to 119 pounds overall, she would adjust her diet so that she stayed at that weight, with her fat decreasing and her muscle increasing by the same amount.

Susan's problem was more extreme than Michael's. He had two options, whereas she only had one. That is, he could have chosen to do only one surgery a day, which would have left him with enough strength and time to recover for the next day. However, that would have cut his income in half, and so was not a realistic option for him. He had to become stronger. Susan, on the other hand, had no energy reserves whatsoever, so she would not have been able to recover even if she spent the whole day in bed. Her only choice was to become stronger.

RELAXATION

After years of training clients, we observed with dismay that some of them, even though they exercised and ate properly, were losing muscle instead of fat. We experimented with different approaches to exercising and dieting, but nothing solved the problem. How to reverse this mysterious dynamic occurred to us while we were preparing for the World Weightlifting Championship in 1996.

Because serious weightlifting training causes many fine tears in the muscles, as well as depleting the nervous and hormonal systems, we always followed a training session by sitting in a hot tub to repair those muscles and restore those systems. Nevertheless, although we relaxed our bodies in this way, we were still stressed mentally as we thought about the upcoming competition, and that stress prevented us from recovering fully.

Searching for ways to relax our minds, we found that meditation relaxed us the most. At the same time, over a period of weeks, as we studied our daily journals, where we recorded our own measurements, we noticed that we were losing fat while gaining muscle mass. Since the only change in our routines was the addition of meditation, we concluded that meditation must have something to do with the loss of fat.

In analyzing this phenomenon, we thought it might be related to the parasympathetic nervous system. The body has two nervous systems: the sympathetic, which controls action, and the

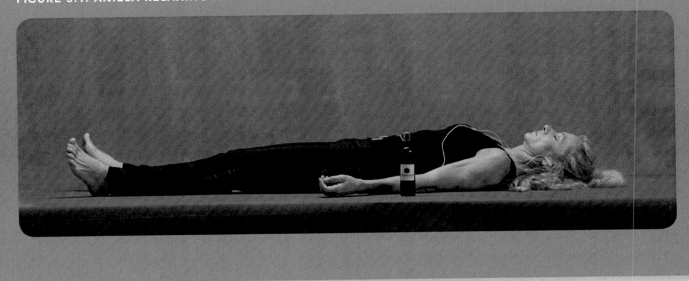

parasympathetic, which controls recovery from action. The first system uses adenosine triphosphate (ATP) as energy, which helps one to lift; the second system uses fat as energy which helps one to recover. Therefore, the more relaxed we are after we exercise, the more fat we burn.

Athletes use ATP during explosive movements because it is the fastest energy fuel provided by the body. When ATP is depleted, the body burns sugar for energy, then muscle, and finally fat.

Thus, the body burns fat when it is either exhausted or relaxed. We didn't want to exhaust our clients, but to relax them. In the context of exercise, there are many ways to relax, such as getting a massage or spending time in a sauna, hot tub, or steam room. But these relax the body without necessarily relaxing the mind. To relax both the body and the mind, without the help of other people or complicated equipment, one need only practice daily meditation. We have found, after much experimentation, that this works best combined with aromatherapy and meditative music. For these, a bottle of essential oil and an iPod* or CD player are all one needs. In The Happy Body program, we use lavender oil and Jules Massenet's "Meditation from Thais" (specifically, the version performed by the Budapest Philharmonic Orchestra) to relax our clients after they have completed their exercise routines (Figure 5.1).

When they have used aroma therapy and music for several weeks, our clients not only lose fat and gain muscle, but they also become calmer, more rational, and more pleasant.

Thus, in any exercise program, mental relaxation is just as important as the physical activity. Furthermore, relaxation is just as important outside the context of exercise. We have found, for example, that whenever our clients are nervous or tense, they only have to play the Massenet piece and, like a mantra, it immediately relaxes them.

REJUVENATION

Rejuvenation is the other essential element of recovery. But it can only make you as youthful as you were yesterday. You cannot improve your youthfulness without knowing when and how to rest. The more work you do, and the more intense it is, the more time you need to take to rejuvenate.

For example, sprinters who run 100 meters in 10 seconds may need 8 minutes to fully recover for the next race, whereas the same runners, warming up and completing 100 meters in 15 seconds, may need only 3 minutes to fully recover. This principle applies to performers of any kind. Pianists, for instance, cannot practice indefinitely for a recital. They need to know when to rest and for how long.

In fact, everyone is a performer. To be alive is to perform. But if we work too much and rest too little, we exhaust ourselves, and if we work too little and rest too much, we deteriorate.

The question is, how do you know how much to perform and how much to rest? The easiest way is to observe how you feel when you wake up in the morning. If you get out of bed feeling excited about the day and eager to accomplish things, you are fine. But if you get out of bed without enthusiasm and energy for the day, your life is out of balance. So the key to rejuvenation is how you feel first thing in the morning.

RECOVERY AND RELAXATION DURING EXERCISE

Up to now, we have been talking about recovery and relaxation after exercise. However, in The Happy Body program, we also recover and relax while we exercise. That is, every repetition in the program has three parts: 1. inhaling, 2. moving while holding the breath, and 3. exhaling. It is during this third part that we recover and relax. As we exhale, we are letting go mentally of the previous repetition and releasing the tension we created and developed during the movement. The mental release during exhalation can be thought of as a moment of micro-meditation. This breathing technique, which we adapted from Olympic weightlifting, improves the quality of each repetition by incorporating rest into the activity.

In fact, this breathing technique, which is not used by any other fitness program, helps people to simultaneously achieve all six Standards of Youthfulness. For example, with the exhalation that follows every movement, our clients completely relax every muscle fiber in their bodies. Over time, this elongates the muscles and makes our clients more limber, so that they ultimately achieve The Happy Body Standard of Flexibility.

While performing The Happy Body exercises, our clients create an inner observer, especially as they exhale. Like dancers or gymnasts, they develop a heightened awareness of where they are in space and time and of which parts of their bodies are in or out of balance. Gradually, this awareness contributes to achieving The Happy Body Standard of Good Posture.

When our clients are working to achieve The Happy Body Standard of Ideal Body Weight, they want to lose fat, not muscle. Endurance programs, which involve continuous training, cause the loss of muscle because they do not provide for rest between repetitions. Our program, on the other hand, which is a form of interval training, promotes the loss of fat precisely because it provides for rest between repetitions.

Most of our clients—more than 99% of them, in fact—come to us not only needing to lose fat but to gain muscle. The relaxation and the rest that we incorporate into every repetition in the exercises allow muscles to recover and repair themselves, which stimulates them to increase in size. Thus, our interval training promotes The Happy Body Standard of Leanness by correcting the proportion of muscle to fat.

With their bigger muscles, our clients become stronger, but they have not yet fully achieved The Happy Body Standard of Strength. To do that, they must increase the production of the hormones in the brain that stimulate muscle fibers. During every exhalation, the brain has a moment to restore the level of those hormones. Over time, as our clients lift heavier and heavier weights, they elevate the level of those hormones as they relax.

Finally, our clients can have big, strong muscles that have not yet achieved The Happy Body Standard of Speed. To do that, they must accelerate the production and delivery of those hormones that stimulate muscle fibers. Over time, as our clients lift their weights faster and faster, they accelerate the production and delivery of those hormones as they relax.

Far Better and More Efficient

Steven F. Kanter (60-year-old doctor)

Although I had not had a trainer since high school, I decided to work with Jerzy because most of my problems had come from overdoing sports and aerobic training. At its worst this habit had lead to a serious case of heat stroke (my urine turned jet black), orthopedic injuries, numerous 'minor' overuse injuries, and muscle cramping.

Since becoming a physician in 1973, I followed the medical literature relating to exercise, fitness, weight, and health. I had generally practiced conventional wisdom by becoming aerobically fit with only minor strength training.

The best shape I was ever in had been during high school when I wrestled in the 127-pound weight class. Motivated by my love of sports and my family's history of heart disease, I had continued to play multiple sports and stay aerobically fit by running, swimming, and bicycling. I also maintained a fairly healthy Mediterranean style diet. Then, two weeks before turning 57, I underwent a 13-hour radical back and pelvic surgery that removed a large, cancerous tumor as well as my coccyx and most of my sacrum.

During and after my recovery, I swam about a mile a day — 5 days a week — performed calisthenics and curls every other day, and I resumed playing golf 2 to 4 times a week.

Seven months after my radical surgery, I fractured a vertebra on a difficult golf swing. After 4 months of unsuccessful bed rest, I had surgery to repair the fracture, which included the insertion of two large titanium screws. Three months after that surgery, I was in a collision that caused my car to careen into a traffic pole at about 40 mph. My car was totaled. Although my vertebra screws held, I developed worsening pelvic and back pain, and the neurological recovery I had experienced since my radical surgery was completely wiped out.

After several months, I gradually tried to exercise again. My wife at the time, who had unsuccessfully tried a long list of other programs, had begun to use Jerzy as a trainer. I observed how she was able to change her body shape using The Happy Body program. In part because Jerzy had personal experience with a significant spine injury, I met with him and reviewed with him how a modified program might help me improve my physical functioning and help reduce my pain. Additionally, although my weight was in the normal range, my percentage of body fat was high and we both felt I could benefit from being leaner.

Due to my injuries, Jerzy was adamant that I not overdo my exercising; I had to agree to never do more than what he prescribed for me. Jerzy's firsthand knowledge of rehabilitation from a serious spine injury, and his holistic approach (exercise, proper nutrition, relaxation, and paying attention to your body's reactions to all three) made more sense to me than what I had been doing. I have not experienced any injuries or setbacks due to the program.

What I have experienced is that The Happy Body works far better and takes less time than when I maintained a very high level of aerobic fitness. After a very cautious beginning, I am now in the best shape I've been in since I wrestled 45 years ago. The Happy Body program has made an invaluable improvement in my physical well-being, fitness, physique, and joy in life!

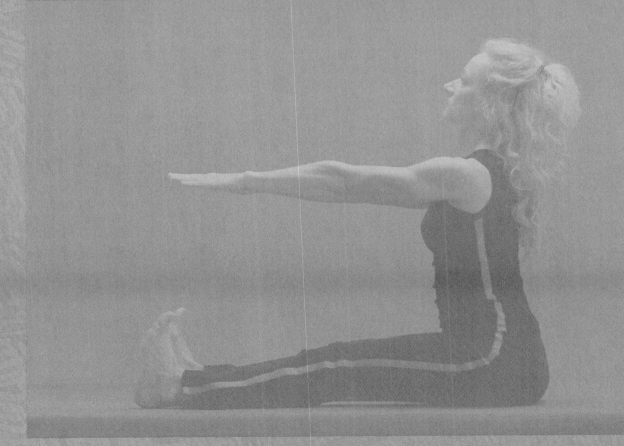

DESIGNING THE HAPPY BODY

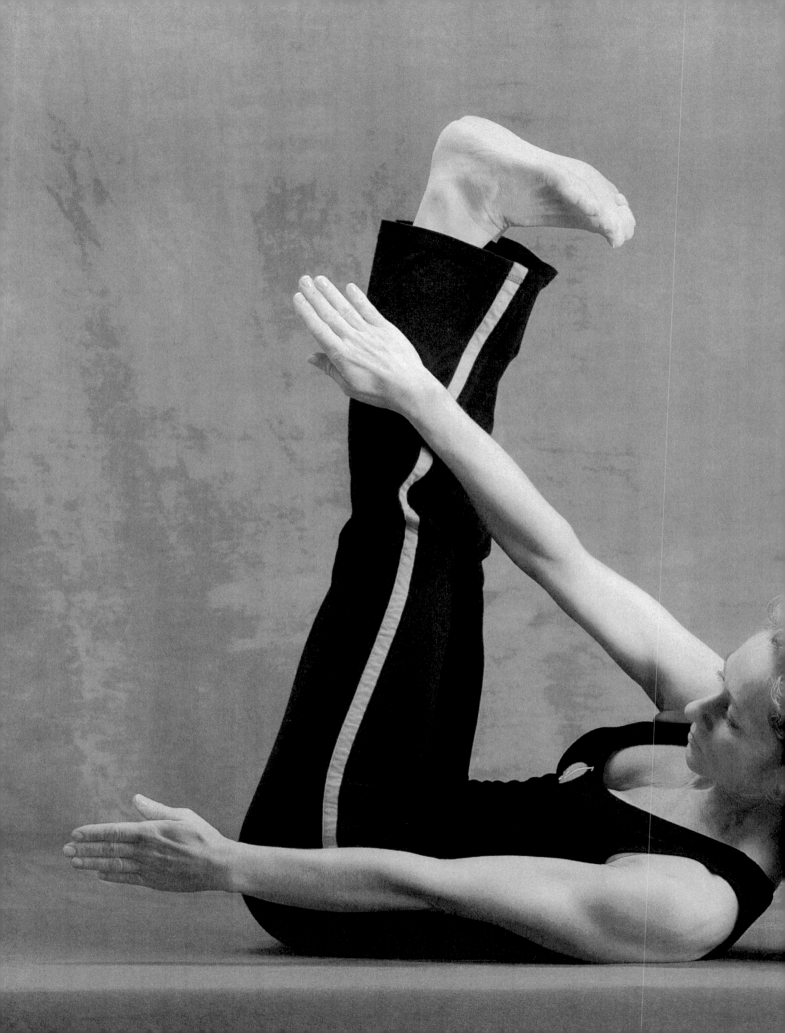

PART 2

COUNTING TIME & POUNDS

THE IDEAL BODY

To achieve a happy body, you first have to calculate the time it will take you to reach your Ideal Body Weight Proportions—that is, the ideal proportions between your height, weight, muscle, and fat, depending on your gender. Then you have to design an eating program to control your metabolic rate. Next, you have to learn the exercises to achieve the Standards of Youthfulness. Finally, you have to master the art of recovery.

WEEK 1

CALCULATING YOUR IDEAL BODY WEIGHT PROPORTIONS

Step 1

You begin by determining what your Ideal Body Weight Proportions are, which you will find by your height in Table 6.1 (for females) and Table 6.2 (for males).

The examples given for this step, and for all subsequent ones throughout this book, will be for a woman who is 5'2" tall. The ideal proportions for such a woman are:

Ideal Body Weight: 110.0 lbs
Ideal fat weight: 14.3 lbs
Ideal muscle weight: 95.7 lbs

Enter your Ideal Body Weight Proportions:

Your Ideal Body Weight: _____ lbs

Your ideal fat weight: _____ lbs

Your ideal muscle weight: _____ lbs

TABLE 6.1: IDEAL FEMALE BODY WEIGHT PROPORTIONS (13% FAT)			
Height	**Weight** (pounds)	**Fat** (pounds)	**Muscle** (pounds)
4'10"	98	12.7	85.3
4'11"	101	13.1	87.9
5'0"	104	13.5	90.5
5'1"	107	13.9	93.1
5'2"	**110**	**14.3**	**95.7**
5'3"	113	14.7	98.3
5'4"	116	15.1	100.9
5'5"	119	15.5	103.5
5'6"	122	15.9	106.1
5'7"	125	16.3	108.7
5'8"	128	16.6	111.4
5'9"	131	17.2	114.8
5'10"	134	17.6	117.4
5'11"	137	17.9	120.1
6'0"	140	18.5	123.5
6'1"	143	18.9	126.1
6'2"	147	19.6	130.4
6'3"	150	20.2	134.8
6'4"	153	20.8	139.2

CHAPTER 6: COUNTING TIME AND POUNDS

TABLE 6.2: IDEAL MALE BODY WEIGHT PROPORTIONS (10% FAT)			
Height	**Weight** (pounds)	**Fat** (pounds)	**Muscle** (pounds)
4'10"	110	11.0	99.0
4'11"	115	11.5	103.5
5'0"	120	12.0	108.0
5'1"	125	12.5	112.5
5'2"	130	13.0	117.0
5'3"	135	13.5	121.5
5'4"	140	14.0	126.0
5'5"	145	14.5	130.5
5'6"	150	15.0	135.0
5'7"	155	15.5	139.5
5'8"	160	16.0	146.0
5'9"	165	16.5	148.5
5'10"	170	17.0	153.0
5'11"	175	17.5	157.5
6'0"	180	18.0	162.0
6'1"	185	18.5	166.5
6'2"	190	19.0	171.0
6'3"	195	19.5	175.5
6'4"	200	20.0	180.0

Step 2

After you have determined your Ideal Body Weight Proportions, you calculate your current body weight proportions by weighing yourself and measuring your percentage of body fat. The most accurate way to measure that percentage is with underwater weighing, however that's complicated, expensive, and not readily available. A simpler but still fairly accurate method is to measure the skin folds on your body—for that all you need are your fingers and a caliper. But we have simplified it even further. All you need are your fingers and a ruler. The process is slightly different for males and females, because a female's triceps must be measured from behind by another person. For both genders, you take three measurements of your skin folds (Figure 6.1), add these measurements together, and then locate your body fat percentage in Table 6.3.

FIGURE 6.1: MEASURING THE SKIN FOLDS ON YOUR BODY

FEMALES

MALES

TRICEPS SKIN FOLD

CHEST SKIN FOLD

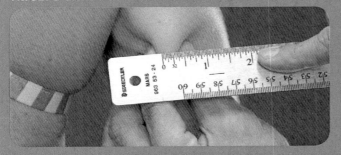
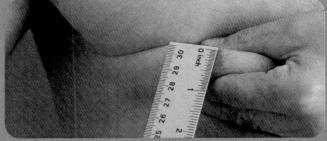

SIDE OF ABDOMEN

ABDOMEN SKIN FOLD

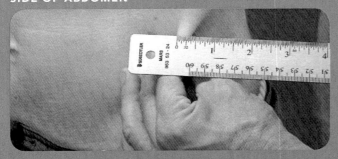
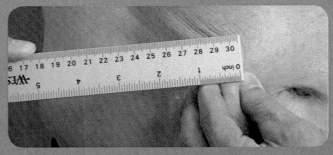

THIGH SKIN FOLD

THIGH SKIN FOLD

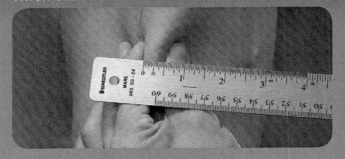
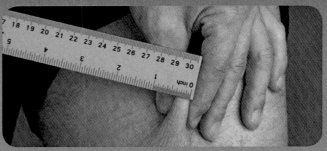

TABLE 6.3: PERCENTAGE OF BODY FAT BY SKIN FOLD MEASUREMENTS

Total (inches)	Female Body Fat (percentage)	Male Body Fat (percentage)
1 $\frac{3}{16}$	13	10
1 $\frac{3}{8}$	15	11
1 $\frac{9}{16}$	17	12
1 $\frac{3}{4}$	19	13.5
2	21	15
2 $\frac{3}{16}$	22.5	16.5
2 $\frac{3}{8}$	24	18
2 $\frac{9}{16}$	26.5	19.5
2 $\frac{3}{4}$	27	21
3	28.5	22.5
3 $\frac{3}{16}$	30	23
3 $\frac{3}{8}$	31.5	24.5
3 $\frac{9}{16}$	33	26
3 $\frac{3}{4}$	34	27
4	35	28
4 $\frac{3}{16}$	36	29
4 $\frac{3}{8}$	37	30
4 $\frac{9}{16}$	38	31
4 $\frac{3}{4}$	39	32
5	40	33
5 $\frac{3}{16}$	41	34
5 $\frac{3}{8}$	42	35

As an example, let's say if you are a female whose three measurements are 2 $^5/_{16}$", 2 $^1/_{16}$", and $^{11}/_{16}$", your total is 5 $^1/_{16}$". If you fall between the given numbers in Table 5, use the percentage closest to your number. If your total is 5 $^1/_{16}$", you are closest to 5". That would mean your body is 40% fat.

Step 3

Next, calculate how many pounds of fat and muscle you have today by following this equation:

Your body fat today = body weight x body fat %.

If you are a female who weighs 146 pounds, and your body fat is 40% (.40), then your body fat is 58.4 pounds as in the following equation:

146 x .40 = 58.4

What's remaining is muscle. For the same 146 pound woman it looks like this:

146 – 58.4 = 87.6

Step 4

Determine whether you have too much or too little fat and muscle.

For example, if you weigh 146 pounds, and your Ideal Body Weight is 110 pounds, you are overweight. If your fat is 58.4 pounds, and your ideal fat is 14.3 pounds, you have too much fat (44.1 pounds). Calculate it like this:

58.4 – 14.3 = 44.1

If your muscle is 87.6 pounds, and your ideal muscle is 95.7 pounds, you have too little muscle (8.1 pounds):

95.7 – 87.6 = 8.1

Step 5

The final step is to determine your body type in Table 6.4. Then you can follow the program for that specific type, which will transform you into Type 1 (Ideal Body Type) in a measurable amount of time.

Bye-Bye Body Fat

Reno Wilson (31-year-old actor)

I started The Happy Body program with Jerzy and Aniela to see how having a ripped physique might affect my acting career. In only eight weeks, I went from 16% body fat down to 8%! In the next four weeks, I lost another 4%. Not only was I lean, but many more acting offers began to come in.

A year after I started the program, I got a role that required me to do a shower scene and be even more "ripped" than I already was. So Jerzy and Aniela made a few modifications in my program, which got me down to 3% fat in only six weeks. Then, for the last week before I had to do the scene, they gave me special instructions, just like the ones they follow during the last week before they compete in Olympic weightlifting championships. That got me down to 2% body fat in eight days. I was amazed at how good I looked!

Now I work steadily, my income has more than doubled, and the simple and effective Happy Body exercises and diet are a regular part of my lifestyle, even when I'm on the road.

TABLE 6.4: THIRTEEN POSSIBLE BODY TYPES FOR A 5'2" FEMALE						
Type Number (pounds)	Fat Content	Muscle Content	Weight (pounds)	Body (%)	Fat (pounds)	Muscle
Ideal Weight						
1	ideal	ideal	110	13	14.3	95.7
2	too little	too much	110	5	5.5	104.5
3	too much	too little	110	30	33	77
Overweight						
4	ideal	too much	143	10	14.3	128.7
5	too much	ideal	145	34	49.3	95.7
6	too much	too much	166	35	58.1	107.9
7	**too much**	**too little**	**146**	**42**	**61.32**	**84.68**
8	too little	too much	125	8	10	115
Underweight						
9	ideal	too little	100	14.3	14.3	85.7
10	too little	too little	90	10	9	81
11	too much	too little	100	30	30	70
12	too little	ideal	104	8	8.3	95.7
13	too little	too much	104	5	5.2	98.8.

Now that you know your body type, we will show you how to calculate the time it will take to achieve your Ideal Body Weight and Ideal Body Weight Proportions. We will also show you how to proceed with losing or gaining fat or muscle, and how to maintain your Ideal Body Weight Proportions once you achieve them.

CALCULATING THE TIME TO REACH YOUR IDEAL BODY WEIGHT PROPORTIONS

In all the years that we have worked with clients, the first thing they want to know, after they calculate their ideal body goals, is "How long will it take me?" At first, we could only make educated guesses. But our clients, and we ourselves, wished we had a more precise way to make this calculation.

We researched if anyone else had the answer to this problem, but everyone seemed to be making approximate guesses, just like us. That led us to collect weekly data about our clients, and eventually we were able to determine certain averages.

For example, we discovered that our clients were losing fat at a rate of 1% of their Ideal Body Weight every week. Those people usually needed to gain muscle at the same time, and we noticed that they were doing so at a rate of 0.2% of their Ideal Body Weight every week—that is, five times slower than they lost fat.

A small percentage of our clients arrived at our studio needing to gain fat, and we learned from them that they gained fat at the same rate that other people lost fat—namely, at 1% of their Ideal Body Weight every week (Table 6.5).

Finally, a tiny percentage of our clients arrived at our studio needing to lose muscle, and we learned that they lost it roughly twice as fast as people lose or gain fat—namely, at 2% of their Ideal Body Weight every week.

Before you calculate your rates of loss or gain, determine your Ideal Body Weight for your height from Table 6.1 (females) or Table 6.2 (males), pages 75 and 76.

Example
Our 5'2" female has an Ideal Body Weight of 110 pounds. Therefore, her rate of fat loss or gain per week is 1.1 pounds:

$$110 \times .01 = 1.1$$

Her rate of muscle loss is 2.2 pounds per week:

$$110 \times .02 = 2.2$$

Her rate of muscle gain is 0.22 pounds per week:

$$110 \times .002 = 0.22$$

These are her four personal rates of loss or gain. With these numbers, she is now equipped to calculate how long it will take her to achieve her Ideal Body Weight Proportions. Since she is Body Type 7, she will plug these numbers into the formulas for that type.

TABLE 6.5: WEEKLY RATES OF LOSING AND GAINING	
Losing fat	1% (.01) of Ideal Body Weight
Gaining fat	1% (.01) of Ideal Body Weight
Losing muscle	2% (.02) of Ideal Body Weight
Gaining muscle	0.2% (.002) of Ideal Body Weight

The Confidence To Know

Kelly Walsh (42-year-old career counselor)

I was living in a very unhappy body. I hated seeing myself in pictures. My clothes didn't fit. I'd never get in the pool with my young children because I wouldn't put on a bathing suit. More seriously, I had high cholesterol and a family history of heart disease. I knew I needed to lose some weight if I wanted to be around to see my kids grow up, but I'd tried unsuccessfully for years.

Last summer, a friend told me about Jerzy and Aniela and gave me Jerzy's email.

The first meeting was emotionally rough. I went into it thinking that if I lost about 25 pounds I'd be happy. Jerzy took my measurements and pictures from all angles in a bathing suit and told me I should lose 60 pounds. Boy, was I shocked! I didn't think it was realistic to lose that much weight. A funny thing happened, though: the pounds started coming off, and that goal no longer seemed so far-fetched.

The Happy Body diet is really quite easy to follow. I've come to love my hemp bread with egg whites in the mornings and don't miss the old cereal, bagels, muffins I used to eat. But you do have to follow the whole program. It's all scientifically based, and if you follow their plan you absolutely lose weight.

The exercise component of their program was a little harder for me. I have always loved doing cardio workouts and was doing a cardio "boot camp" when I started with them. They strongly discouraged me from continuing with it. I quit, and as the months went on, I heard more and more about friends with early arthritis, back pains, and knee problems from overuse and training. I came to accept what the Gregoreks teach about strength, flexibility, and creating a Happy Body as opposed to a broken, tired one.

At certain intervals, Jerzy again takes measurements and bathing suit pictures and has you compare your latest pictures side by side with your old ones. It's amazing to look at the differences and a great motivation to keep going.

As of now I've lost 23 pounds, and I definitely feel much better than when I started. I still have a ways to go, but I finally have a solid plan and the confidence that I can and will do it. I can't wait to buy new clothes when I reach my goal. Thank you Jerzy and Aniela.

THIRTEEN BODY TYPES

O n the following pages, you will find all thirteen body types. Find your body type, as you determined on page 80, and plug your own personal numbers in to find your weekly rates of loss and gain to achieve your Ideal Body. Then go to Chapter 7 to design your eating program.

BODY TYPE 1
The Happy Body

Weight	Fat	Muscle
Ideal	Ideal	Ideal

Example

If you are a 5'2" female, you weigh 110 pounds, your fat is 13% (.13), your fat weighs14.3 pounds:

110 x .13 = 14.3

Your muscle weighs 95.7 pounds:

110 – 14.3 = 95.7

Since you already have Ideal Body Weight Proportions, according to The Happy Body standards, you can skip the nutrition plan and go straight to the exercise program to begin achieving the other Standards of Youthfulness.

BODY TYPE 2
The Gymnast

Weight	Fat	Muscle
Ideal	Too Little	Too Much

Example

If you are a 5'2" female, and you weigh 110 pounds, and your fat is 5% (.05), then your fat weighs 5.5 pounds:

$$110 \times .05 = 5.5$$

Your muscle weighs 104.5 pounds:

$$110 - 5.5 = 104.5$$

Step 1

Estimate how many pounds of fat you need to gain and how many pounds of muscle you need to lose.

Since, at 5'2", you should have 14.3 pounds of fat, you must gain 8.8 pounds of fat:

$$14.3 - 5.5 = 8.8$$

You should have 95.7 pounds of muscle, so you must lose 8.8 pounds of muscle:

$$104.5 - 95.7 = 8.8$$

Step 2

Estimate how many pounds of fat you will gain per week and how many pounds of muscle you will lose per week. At 1% (.01) of your Ideal Body Weight every week, you will gain 1.1 pounds of fat per week:

$$110 \times .01 = 1.1$$

Theoretically, you could lose in muscle 2% (.02) of your Ideal Body Weight every week, in which case you would lose 2.2 pounds of muscle per week:

$$110 \times .02 = 2.2$$

However, since you are already at your Ideal Body Weight, you want to keep your weight constant. If you lost 2.2 pounds of muscle every week, you would lose weight, because you would not gain the same amount of fat. In your case, therefore, you must lose muscle at the same rate that you gain fat—namely, 1.1 pounds per week.

Step 3

Estimate the total time you will need to achieve your Ideal Body Weight Proportions:

$$8.8 \div 1.1 = 8$$

In your case, you will need 8 weeks to achieve your Ideal Body Weight Proportions.

BODY TYPE 3
The Scale Watcher

Weight	Fat	Muscle
Ideal	Too Much	Too Little

Example

If you are a 5'2" female, and you weigh 110 pounds, and your fat is 30% (.3), then your fat weighs 33 pounds:

$$110 \times .3 = 33$$

Your muscle weighs 77 pounds:

$$110 - 33 = 77$$

Step 1

Estimate how many pounds of fat you need to lose and how many pounds of muscle you need to gain.

Since, at 5'2", you should have 14.3 pounds of fat, you must lose 18.7 pounds of fat:

$$33 - 14.3 = 18.7$$

You should have 95.7 pounds of muscle, you must gain 18.7 pounds of muscle:

$$95.70 - 77 = 18.7$$

Step 2

Estimate how many pounds of fat you will lose per week and how many pounds of muscle you will gain per week. At 0.2% (.002) of your Ideal Body Weight per week, you will gain 2.2 pounds of muscle per week:

$$110 \times .002 = 0.22$$

Theoretically, you could lose 1% (.01) in fat of your Ideal Body Weight every week, in which case you would lose 1.1 pounds of fat per week:

$$110 \times .01 = 1.1$$

However, since you are already at your Ideal Body Weight, you want to keep your weight constant. If you lost 1.1 pounds of fat every week, you would lose weight, because you would not gain the same amount of muscle. In your case, therefore, you must lose fat at the same rate that you gain muscle— namely, 0.22 pounds per week.

Step 3

Estimate the total time you will need to achieve your Ideal Body Weight Proportions:

$$18.7 \div 0.22 = 85$$

You will need 85 weeks to achieve your Ideal Body Weight.

BODY TYPE 4
The Lineman

Weight	Fat	Muscle
Too Much	Ideal	Too Much

Example

If you are a 5'2" female, and you weigh 143 pounds and your fat is 10% (0.1), then your fat weighs 14.3 pounds:

$143 \times 0.1 = 14.3$

Your muscle weighs 128.7 pounds:

$143 - 14.3 = 128.7$

Step 1

Estimate how many pounds of muscle you need to lose:

$128.7 - 95.7 = 33$

Since, at 5'2", you should have 95.7 pounds of fat, you must lose 33 pounds of muscle.

Step 2

Estimate how many pounds of muscle you will lose per week: At 2% (.02) of your Ideal Body Weight per week, you will lose 2.2 pounds of muscle per week:

$110 \times .02 = 2.2$

Step 3

Estimate the total time you will need to achieve your Ideal Body Weight Proportions:

$33 \div 2.2 = 15$

Since the weight of your body fat is already ideal, you only need to lose muscle, so you will need 15 weeks to achieve your Ideal Body Weight Proportions.

BODY TYPE 5
The Gym Member

Weight	Fat	Muscle
Too Much	Too Much	Ideal

Example

If you are a 5'2" female, and you weigh 145 pounds and your fat is 34% (.34), then your fat weighs 49.3 pounds:

145 x .34 = 49.3

Your muscle is 95.7 pounds:

145 – 49.3 = 95.7

Step 1

Estimate how many pounds of fat you need to lose:

49.3 – 14.3 = 35

Since, at 5'2", you should have 14.3 pounds of fat, you must lose 35 pounds of fat.

Step 2

Estimate how many pounds of fat you will lose per week: At 1% (.01) of your Ideal Body Weight per week, you will lose 1.1 pounds of fat per week:

110 x .01 = 1.1

Step 3

Estimate the total time you will need to achieve your Ideal Body Weight Proportions:

35 ÷ 1.1 = 31.85

Since your muscle weight is already ideal, you only need to lose fat, so you will need 31.85 weeks to achieve your Ideal Body Weight proportions.

BODY TYPE 6
The Sumo Wrestler

Weight	Fat	Muscle
Too Much	Too Much	Too Much

Example

If you are a 5′2″ female, and you weigh 166 pounds, and your fat is 35% (.35), then your fat weighs 58 pounds:

166 x .35 = 58.1

Your muscle weighs 107.9 pounds:

166 – 58.1 = 107.9

Step 1

Estimate how many pounds of fat you need to lose and how many pounds of muscle you need to lose.

You must lose 43.8 pounds of fat:

58.1 – 14.3 = 43.8

You must lose 12.2 pounds of muscle:

107.9 – 95.7 = 12.2

Step 2

Estimate how many pounds of fat and how many pounds of muscle you will lose per week. At 2% (.02) of your Ideal Body Weight per week, you will lose 2.2 pounds of muscle per week:

110 x .02 = 2.2

At 1% (.01) of your Ideal Body Weight per week, you will lose 1.1 pounds of fat per week:

110 x .01 = 1.1

Step 3

Estimate the total time you will need to achieve your Ideal Body Weight Proportions:

43.8 ÷ 1.1 = 39.82

Since it is best to stay strong while you are losing weight, it is preferable to lose that weight first in fat and then in muscle. Therefore, since you will be losing fat first, it will take you 39.82 weeks to lose 43.8 pounds of fat.

Next, to lose 12.2 pounds of muscle, you will need an additional 5.55 weeks to achieve your Ideal Body Weight Proportions:

12.2 ÷ 2.2 = 5.55

Thus, you will need a total of 45.37 weeks to achieve your Ideal Body Weight Proportions:

39.82 + 5.55 = 45.37

BODY TYPE 7
The Sitter

Weight	Fat	Muscle
Too Much	Too Much	Too Little

Example

If you are a 5'2" female, and you weigh 146 pounds and your fat is 42% (.42), then your fat weighs 61.32 pounds:

$$146 \times .42 = 61.32$$

Your muscle weighs 84.68 pounds:

$$146 - 61.32 = 84.68$$

Step 1

Estimate how many pounds of fat you need to lose and how many pounds of muscle you need to gain.

You must lose 47.02 pounds of fat:

$$61.32 - 14.30 = 47.02$$

You must gain 11.02 pounds of muscle:

$$95.70 - 84.68 = 11.02$$

Step 2

Estimate how many pounds of fat you will lose per week and how many pounds of muscle you will gain per week. At 1% (.01) of your Ideal Body Weight per week, you will lose 1.1 pounds of fat per week:

$$110 \times .01 = 1.1$$

At 0.2% (.002) of your Ideal Body Weight per week, you will gain .22 pounds of muscle per week:

$$110 \times .002 = 0.22$$

Step 3

Estimate how much time it will take you to achieve your Ideal Body Weight Proportions.

It will take you 42.74 weeks to lose 47.02 pounds of fat:

$$47.02 \div 1.1 = 42.74$$

And it will take you 50.09 weeks to gain 11.02 pounds of muscle:

$$11.02 \div .22 = 50.09$$

Since the time to lose fat is shorter than the time to gain muscle, the latter is the time you will need to achieve your Ideal Body Weight Proportions. (The bigger number will always be the time it will take to achieve your Ideal Body Weight Proportions.)

BODY TYPE 8
The Bodybuilder

Weight	Fat	Muscle
Too Much	Too Little	Too Much

Example

If you are a 5'2" female, and you weigh 125 pounds and your fat is 8% (.08), then your fat weighs 10 pounds:

125 x .08= 10

Your muscle weighs 115 pounds:

125 – 10 = 115

Step 1

Estimate how many pounds of fat you need to gain and how many pounds of muscle you need to lose.

You must gain 4.3 pounds of fat:

14.3 – 10 = 4.3

You must lose 19.3 pounds of muscle:

115 – 95.70 = 19.3

Step 2

Estimate how many pounds of fat you will gain per week and how many pounds of muscle you will lose per week. At 2% (.02) of your Ideal Body Weight per week, you will lose 2.2 pounds of muscle per week:

110 x .02 = 2.2

At 1% (.01) of your Ideal Body Weight per week, you will gain 1.1 pounds of fat per week:

110 x .01 = 1.1

Step 3

Estimate how much time it will take you to achieve your Ideal Body Weight Proportions.

It will take you 3.9 weeks to gain 4.3 pounds of fat:

4.3 ÷ 1.1 = 3.9

It will take you 8.77 weeks to lose 19.3 pounds of muscle:

19.3 ÷ 2.2 = 8.77

Since the time to gain fat is shorter than the time to lose muscle, the latter is the time you will need to achieve your Ideal Body Weight Proportions. (The bigger number will always be the time it will take to achieve your Ideal Body Weight Proportions.)

BODY TYPE 9
The Fashion Model

Weight	Fat	Muscle
Too Little	Ideal	Too Little

Example

If you are a 5'2" female, and you weigh 100 pounds and your fat is 14.3% (0.143), then your fat weighs 14.3 pounds:

100 x 0.143 = 14.3

Your muscle weighs 85.7 pounds:

100 – 14.3 = 85.7

Step 1

Estimate how many pounds of muscle you need to gain:

95.7 – 85.7 = 10

You must gain 10 pounds of muscle.

Step 2

Estimate how many pounds of muscle you will gain per week. At 0.2% (.002) of your Ideal Body Weight per week, you will gain .22 pounds of muscle per week:

110 x .002 = 0.22

Step 3

Estimate how much time it will take you to achieve your Ideal Body Weight Proportions:

10 ÷.22 = 45.45

It will take you 45.45 weeks to gain 10 pounds of muscle.

BODY TYPE 10
The Twig

Weight	Fat	Muscle
Too Little	Too Little	Too Little

Example
If you are a 5'2" female, and you weigh 90 pounds and your fat is 10% (0.1), then your fat weighs 9 pounds:

$$90 \times 0.1 = 9$$

Your muscle weighs 81 pounds:

$$90 - 9 = 81$$

Step 1
Estimate how many pounds of fat and muscle you need to gain.

You must gain 5.3 pounds of fat:

$$14.3 - 9 = 5.3$$

You must gain 14.7 pounds of muscle:

$$95.7 - 81 = 14.7$$

Step 2
Estimate how many pounds of fat and muscle you will gain per week. At 0.2% (.002) of your Ideal Body Weight per week, you will gain .22 pounds of muscle per week:

$$110 \times .002 = 0.22$$

At 1% (.01) of your Ideal Body Weight per week, you will gain 1.1 pounds of fat per week:

$$110 \times .01 = 1.1$$

Step 3
Estimate how much time it will take you to achieve your Ideal Body Weight Proportions:

$$5.3 \div 1.1 = 4.82$$

It will take you 4.82 weeks to gain 5.3 pounds of fat.

And it will take you 66.82 weeks to gain 14.7 pounds of muscle:

$$14.7 \div .22 = 66.82$$

Since the time to gain fat is shorter than the time to gain muscle, the latter is the time you will need to achieve your Ideal Body Weight Proportions. (The bigger number will always be the time it will take to achieve your Ideal Body Weight Proportions.)

BODY TYPE 11
The Dieter

Weight	Fat	Muscle
Too Little	Too Much	Too Little

Example
If you are a 5'2" female, and you weigh 100 pounds and your fat is 30% (.3), then your fat weighs 30 pounds:

$100 \times 0.3 = 30$

Your muscle weighs 70 pounds:

$100 - 30 = 70$

Step 1
Estimate how many pounds of fat you need to lose and how many pounds of muscle you need to gain.

You must lose 15.7 pounds of fat:

$30 - 14.3 = 15.7$

You must gain 10 pounds of muscle:

$95.7 - 70 = 25.7$

Step 2
Estimate how many pounds of fat you will lose and how many pounds of muscle you will gain per week. At 1% (.01) of your Ideal Body Weight per week, you will lose 1.1 pounds of fat per week:

$110 \times .01 = 1.1$

At 0.2% (.002) of your Ideal Body Weight per week, you will gain .22 pounds of muscle per week:

$110 \times .002 = 0.22$

Step 3
Estimate how much time it will take you to achieve your Ideal Body Weight Proportions:

$15.7 \div 1.1 = 14.27$

It will take you 14.27 weeks to lose 15.7 pounds of fat.

It will take you 116.82 weeks to gain 25.7 pounds of muscle:

$25.7 \div 0.22 = 116.82$

Since the time to lose fat is shorter than the time to gain muscle, the latter is the time you will need to achieve your Ideal Body Weight Proportions. (The bigger number will always be the time it will take to achieve your Ideal Body Weight Proportions.)

BODY TYPE 12
The Dancer

Weight	Fat	Muscle
Too Little	Too Little	Ideal

Example

If you are a 5'2" female, and you weigh 104 pounds and your fat is 8% (.08), then your fat weighs 8.3 pounds:

$104 \times 0.08 = 8.3$

Your muscle weighs 95.7 pounds:

$104 - 8.3 = 95.7$

Step 1

Estimate how many pounds of fat you need to gain:

$14.3 - 8.3 = 6$

You must gain 6 pounds of fat.

Step 2

Estimate how many pounds of fat you will gain per week. At 1% (.01) of your Ideal Body Weight per week, you will gain 1.1 pounds of fat per week:

$110 \times .01 = 1.1$

Step 3

Estimate the total time you will need to achieve your Ideal Body Weight Proportions:

$6 \div 1.1 = 5.45$

You will need 5.45 weeks to achieve your Ideal Body Weight Proportions.

BODY TYPE 13
The Mountain Climber

Weight	Fat	Muscle
Too Little	Too Little	Too Much

Example
If you are a 5'2" female, and you weigh 104 pounds and your fat is 5% (0.05), then your fat weighs 5.2 pounds:

$104 \times 0.05 = 5.2$

Your muscle weighs 98.8 pounds:

$104 - 5.2 = 98.8$

Step 1
Estimate how many pounds of fat you need to gain and how many pounds of muscle you need to lose.

You must gain 9.1 pounds of fat:

$14.3 - 5.2 = 9.1$

You must lose 3.1 pounds of muscle:

$98.8 - 95.7 = 3.1$

Step 2
Estimate how many pounds of fat you will gain per week and how many pounds of muscle you will lose per week. At 1% (.01) of your Ideal Body Weight per week, you will gain 1.1 pounds of fat per week:

$110 \times .01 = 1.1$

At 2% (.02) of your Ideal Body Weight per week, you will lose 2.2 pounds of muscle per week:

$110 \times .2 = 2.2$

Step 3
Estimate the total time you will need to achieve your Ideal Body Weight Proportions:

$9.1 \div 1.1 = 8.27$

You will need 8.27 weeks to gain 9.1 pounds of fat.

You will need 1.4 weeks to lose 3.1 pounds of muscle:

$3.1 \div 2.2 = 1.4$

Since the time to gain fat is longer than the time to lose muscle, the former is the time you will need to achieve your Ideal Body Weight Proportions. (The bigger number will always be the time it will take to achieve your Ideal Body Weight Proportions.)

Going Against the Pack

Susan Myers (58-year-old community volunteer)

Jerzy and Aniela have changed my life. As with so many, after the age of 40 I had gradually added a fair amount of weight to my slight frame. In denial, I had even lied on my driver's license, subtracting 10 pounds because it made me feel better. At some point, I realized, I had to get help.

When I began the The Happy Body program, Jerzy asked me to do two things: overcome my reluctance and get on the scale, because it was important to know the truth. I also had to put on a bikini and be photographed from the front, the back, and — God, help me — the side.

I somehow made it through that first appointment and decided to pursue the program 100%. Within eight months, I'd lost 26 pounds. Not long after that, I had touched down on the goal weight of 110 — a weight I thought I could never see again, and one I thought Aniela and Jerzy had been crazy to expect I could achieve.

After a while, I committed to memory the whole program—the diet, tools to balance your glycemic index, and The Happy Body series of exercises—and did them automatically each day. I loved the meditation music I listened to after doing my weights, as well. I calmed down and lost weight. I started to feel a new confidence, and I was amazed to see the changes in my body and in my life. People around me started noticing, too. Instead of just going with the pack, I had committed to something that forced me to separate from it. For instance, I eat very differently from everyone else. My bread, almond butter, and bars have seen Norway, Papua New Guinea, and New York, among others. Where I go, they go.

Once I got down to my maintenance weight and shape, I started experimenting with eating out and splurging on occasion; on drinking more, having fun, and enjoying life. Jerzy and Aniela have been very supportive and helpful to me as I encountered a whole new world and worked to find the right balance for myself.

It has been four years, and I have maintained my weight and held myself accountable to my goals. I will be eternally grateful to both Jerzy and Aniela for giving me the tools to succeed. They are wonderful people, and I have learned through my own experience that what they tell me is real. It works. I love how I feel, how I look, and how it has given me a sense of freedom to be in my own body and to feel so much more balanced than I have ever felt before. This is a pursuit of excellence, and I wouldn't want it any other way.

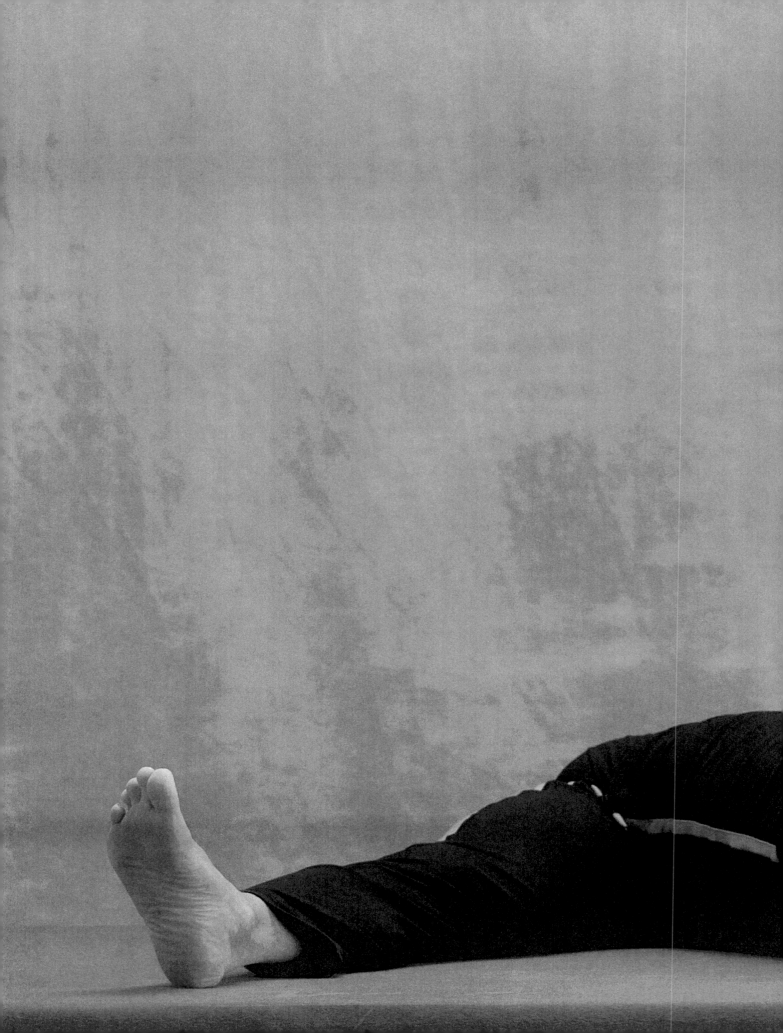

CHAPTER 7

DESIGNING YOUR EATING PROGRAM

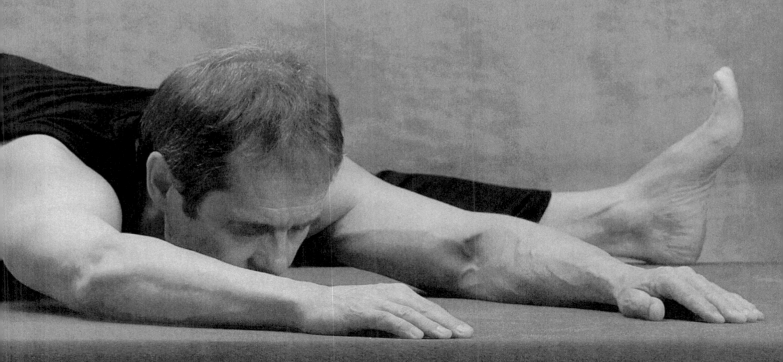

A DIFFERENT KIND OF DIET

This program is not a diet in the normal sense. It is both simpler and more scientific and will give you total control over your body weight and body proportions. It is simpler than regular diets because there are far fewer variables to remember. It is more scientific because it gives you precise formulas to calculate your progress. The simplicity and the precision of the program are what give you the total control, whether you wish to lose, gain, or maintain fat or muscle. Most of all, the program is healthy. Not only will it help you to achieve your Ideal Body, but your blood sugar will be stabilized; your blood pressure will go down; your "good" cholesterol level will go up; your "bad" cholesterol level will go down; your skin will clear; your energy will be high throughout the day, and your sleep will be more restful.

WEEK 1 CONTINUED

First, you must learn which foods are the most efficient for your body. Then, you will learn how to control the volume of your food intake so as to most efficiently reach your goal. Finally, you will learn to schedule your eating on a daily basis with two meals and three snacks.

After you achieve your desired Ideal Body Weight and Ideal Body Weight Proportions, you will learn how to maintain them.

LOSING WEIGHT WITHOUT GIVING UP YOUR FAVORITE FOODS

Most people who lose weight gain it back. This is because, to lose fat, they have had to give up the things they most love to eat and drink: bread, sugar, chocolate, meat, potatoes, rice, beans, coffee, and alcohol. They can do it for a while, but eventually they drift back to their old ways. Our challenge over the years has been to find a program that would enable people to lose fat, and keep it off, without having to give up the things they love. The second thing that people dislike about dieting is counting calories. Our challenge here was to find a simpler, effortless, non-obsessive way to measure and limit food intake without having to use a precise tool such as a scale. Our solutions to both of these problems have proved successful with hundreds of clients.

WHAT TO EAT

From Breakfast to Snack

For most people, breakfast is the unhealthiest meal of the day. Bacon, eggs, sausages, ham, butter, cheese, milk, cream, fruit, juices, breads, bagels, muffins, rolls, donuts, waffles, pancakes, jams, jellies, and cereals are mostly combinations of fat and sugar. Therefore, they provide lots of calories but virtually no protein. However, we keep eating until we get enough protein, so in the process we eat too much fat and sugar. In The Happy Body program, we have eliminated this kind of unhealthy breakfast and replaced it with a healthy snack— one which you choose between health bars, fresh fruit, bread, or yogurt.

Health Bars

You must follow some general guidelines for health bars. They must be nutritionally complete, which means that they should contain protein (10%– 20%), fat (10%–20%), carbohydrates (60%–80%), most vitamins and minerals, and at least 2 grams of fiber for every 100 calories.

Phase 1: While You Are Achieving Your Ideal Body Weight

Since most people are addicted to sugar, we recommend that the first food bars you eat have some sugar content. These include the following brands: Clif Builder's™ (270 calories), Clif® (240 calories), Golean® (270 calories), and Luna™ (170

calories). If you prefer natural and organic foods, the best choices are cold-compressed raw bars. These brands include Attune® (100 calories), Organic Food Bars™ (300 calories), Perfect Foods Bars™ (283 calories), and Lärabar® (190 calories).

When your sugar cravings subside, you can switch to sugarless bars, which include the following brands: Atkins® Advantage™ (240 calories), South Beach Diet™ (210 calories), and thinkThin™ (240 calories).

Phase 2: While You Are Achieving Your Ideal Body Weight Proportions

After you have achieved your Ideal Body Weight, you should start to reduce your consumption of commercial bars except for convenience and occasional cravings. Most of your snacks should now consist of bread, yogurt with fruit, or fresh fruit with nuts.

Phase 3: Maintaining Your Ideal Body Weight Proportions

After you have achieved your Ideal Body Weight Proportions, you should eliminate your consumption of commercial bars and replace them with bars of your own making. These should consist of six ingredients: any kind of nut for crunchiness (30% by calories); dried fruit that still has a little bit of moisture for bonding (50%); dark chocolate with only traces of milk for flavor (5%); protein powder (5%); fiber (5%), and flax seeds (5%). If you decide not to use chocolate or any other ingredient, increase the calorie percentage of fruits. For convenience, your bars should contain in calories 150% of your Ideal Body Weight in pounds. For example, if your Ideal Body Weight is 110 pounds, your bar should contain 165 calories. The best way to do this is to mix 1,650 calories worth of ingredients in a food processor, and then divide the mass into ten equal bars.

Bread

The bread you eat should be organic, whole grain, sprouted and pre-sliced. Furthermore, it should contain 10%–15% protein, 10% fat, 75%–80% carbohydrates, as well as most vitamins and minerals, Omega-3 essential oils, and at least 3 grams of fiber for every 100 calories. It should not contain yeast or processed sugar. After testing many commercial breads, we have had the best results with those manufactured by the Food For Life Baking Company, French Meadow Bakery and Manna Bakery. You can purchase breads from these bakeries in almost any health food store or over the Internet.

Yogurt

Yogurt is a good third alternative for snacks. It aids digestion, has many health benefits, and people like it because they associate it with treats like ice cream. The yogurt should be organic, plain, and non-fat. Check the label for number of calories per ounce, and make adjustments accordingly. If, after you have achieved your Ideal Body Weight, you wish to go to a frozen yogurt parlor, you can add one fruit topping to your portion. Because yogurt lacks fiber, we recommend that you eat it for no more than one snack per day.

Fresh Fruit with Nuts

After you have achieved your Ideal Body Weight, you can reintroduce fresh fruit with nuts as an alternative for a snack, but make sure you stick to your calorie requirements. The proportions should be 80% of fruits and 20% of nuts.

Mixed Snacks

You can mix up your snack types any way you like. Most of our clients like bread in the morning, yogurt or fresh fruit with nuts in the middle of the day, and a bar at the end of the day. If you are traveling, bars are obviously more convenient than bread, yogurt, or fresh fruit with nuts.

Because snacks are high in fiber (with the exception of yogurt) they act like a sponge, absorbing water from your body. Therefore, you should drink at least one glass of water, tea, or coffee with each snack to allow the colon to work properly and to prevent constipation. If you want milk in your tea or coffee, use non-fat milk or soymilk, and be sure that the tea or coffee is dark brown, not beige.

Lunch and Dinner

Your lunch and dinner should contain protein and vegetables. The best sources of animal protein are beef, buffalo, lean pork, wild fish, and seafood. The best sources of plant protein are spinach, tofu, soy beans, broccoli, oat bran, peas, and beans. We recommend eating only limited amounts of chicken, turkey, egg whites, and avoiding fat pork and farm-raised fish altogether, because these foods cause too much inflammation in the body.

The best vegetables are those that are high in fiber, rich in vitamins, and low in sugar. Some vegetables, such as carrots or beets, are high in sugar and are best used as garnishes to enhance the flavor of other vegetables in soups and salads.

Controlling the Volume of Food Intake

If you need to *lose* weight (Body Types 4, 5, 6, 7, 8), the weight of food high in protein you eat in each of your two daily meals should equal in grams 100% of your Ideal Body Weight in pounds, and the vegetables you eat should be double that amount. For each of the three snacks, you should eat in calories 100% of your Ideal Body Weight in pounds.

If you need to *maintain* your weight (Body Types 1, 2, 3), the protein you eat in your two meals should equal in grams 150% of your Ideal Body Weight in pounds, and the vegetables you eat should be double that amount. For each of the three snacks, you should eat in calories 150% of your Ideal Body Weight in pounds.

If you need to *gain* weight (Body Types 9, 10, 11, 12, 13), the protein you eat in your two meals

Steak with Vodka

Don Luskin (51-year-old businessman)

All my life, I've always had the good fortune to find gurus—people who have taught me new ways to think and to live. But by the time I reached the age of 51, I thought the world had run out of them. Then I met the Gregoreks—who may be my best gurus yet.

Gurus aren't just people who can do impossible things. They help others to do impossible things. Aniela and Jerzy certainly qualify after what they've done for me and my wife, Christine. She struggled with her weight for more than twenty years, but nothing helped: diets, pills, nutritionists, endocrinologists all failed. Then she found Aniela and Jerzy. Now, just a few months later, she weighs less and is in better shape and better health than she was the day I married her.

As for me, I've never had a serious weight problem, but I have had a serious fitness problem all my life. I've never played sports or worked out — I just never cared about it —and I was heading slowly but steadily downhill. Then Christine introduced me to Aniela and Jerzy, too. Here are all the impossible things they have helped me do:

- I've lost thirty pounds of fat and gained eleven pounds of muscle, so now I've got a six pack! Before, I never even knew I had muscles there.

- I work out every single day; I never miss even one. What's more impossible is that I like it.

- I eat steak every day and put salt on it.

- I eat hemp bread every day, and I *like* it.

- I eat a pound of vegetables twice a day. Jerzy says I can sometimes substitute vodka for that, but, believe it or not, I've actually come to prefer the vegetables.

should equal in grams 200% of your Ideal Body Weight in pounds, and the vegetables you eat should be double that amount. For each of the three snacks, you should eat in calories 200% of your Ideal Body Weight in pounds.

Example 1: Overweight Types

If you are a 5'2" female, your Ideal Body Weight is 110 pounds. Therefore, you should eat 110 grams of food high in protein and 220 grams of vegetables at each of your two meals, plus 110 calories at each of your three snacks.

Example 2: Ideal Weight Types

If you are a 5'2" female, your Ideal Body Weight is 110 pounds. Therefore, you should eat 165 grams of food high in protein and 330 grams of vegetables at each of your two meals, plus 165 calories at each of your three snacks.

Example 3: Underweight Types

If you are a 5'2" female, your Ideal Body Weight is 110 pounds. Therefore, you should eat 220 grams of food high in protein and 440 grams of vegetables at each of your two meals, plus 220 calories at each of your three snacks.

A simple way to estimate the correct amount of calories in food for lunch or dinner is to use your own hand as a guide. If you need to lose weight, eat the volume of one of your hands in protein and two of your hands in vegetables. If you need to maintain your weight, eat the volume of one and a half of your hands in protein and three of your hands in vegetables. If you need to gain weight, eat the volume of two of your hands in protein and four of your hands in vegetables. (Vegetables include any salad you may eat at lunch or dinner plus the vegetables that accompany the entrée.)

For snacks, you can slice bars by eyeing them, and you can do the same thing with the slices of breads we recommend. To be more precise, you can mark the bar in half, then those two halves in half. So, if you have a bar that is 160 calories, half would be 80, half of that would be 40. If you need to eat 110 calories, it should be very easy for you to see where 110 would be, and where to cut your bar.

If you want to be exact, place your 160 calorie bar on a blank sheet of paper. Divide the bar into 16 even parts. Then you know exactly where to cut your bar so that you have a 110 calorie snack.

When to Eat

Everyone's schedule is a little different. But basically, your eating time every day should occur at 3-hour intervals within a 12-hour period.

The first thing you have to decide is whether you want to base your schedule around lunch or dinner. In either case, those two meals should be six hours apart. Suppose that your job requires you to have lunch every day at noon. In that case, dinner should come at 6:00. On the other hand, if the most important time for you is dinner, and that comes at 8:00, you should have lunch at 2:00. The first snack comes three hours before lunch, the second one comes three hours after lunch, and the third one three hours after dinner.

How to Cope with Eating Out

Obviously, when you are eating at home, you have total control over your food intake. The problem comes when you are eating out, either at a restaurant or someone else's home. Then you must follow certain rules. The first is that you should probably not tell other people that you are following a structured food plan. It is sometimes difficult for others when you change your patterns. We have noticed many of our clients who are at the beginning of the program get derailed by people around them who will challenge them and may unconsciously even want them to fail.

"You eat high sugar bars," they may say. "But sugar is unhealthy! There must be something wrong with that program."

Getting Off the Treadmill

Loren Anderson (21-year-old student)

After three years at college, I came home to San Francisco a lot heavier than I started having gained not only the "freshman 15" but the "freshman 60."

In high school, I had been a very athletic and healthy teenager, but my body changed drastically when I entered a world of college parties and late-night fast-food runs. Because I could not control my eating, I felt as if I could not control my life. At home this past summer I knew something drastically had to change.

At my local gym, before a session with a personal trainer, I warmed up on the treadmill and paged through a magazine. That was where I came across an article about The Happy Body. What caught my attention was that Aniela and Jerzy Gregorek were quoted as saying that endurance training, such as long-distance running or walking on a treadmill, makes people lose muscle, become weaker, and actually get fatter. I got off the treadmill — which I always hated anyway — canceled my appointment, and called the Gregoreks.

For the first time in my adult life, I feel as if I have control over my body and health. The Happy Body is not just a diet and exercise program but a whole lifestyle with meditation and relaxation techniques that help to break old bad habits and establish healthy new ones. For example, I used to turn to food for comfort when I got nervous about a test. Now, I lift my weights and relax with calming music.

I love to cook and eat, but I never feel deprived. I no longer crave cookies or pizza since Aniela and Jerzy guided me to foods that are not only nutritious but delicious.

The only downside to my Happy Body experience has been that my friends have divided into two camps: one side applauded and encouraged me every time I dropped another dress size; the other remained silent or found things to criticize. However, since Jerzy and Aniela had warned me at the beginning about this possibility, I was able to help some of these jealous friends overcome their negativity.

Today, as I approach graduation, I never again will let my body image get in the way of my happiness. Since getting off that treadmill, I feel as if I have the strength to take on the world.

The best policy is to say nothing until they see the progress you've made, and they express the desire to achieve what you have. At that point, you can tell them about The Happy Body program. Of course, some of your friends will be supportive from the beginning, and you can confide in them without any problem.

If you are having dinner at a friend's house and food is served that you don't want to eat but someone asks if anything is wrong, you could say that you have an allergy or a food intolerance, and most people will then leave you alone. Or you could say that you are trying something, but you are not comfortable discussing it yet. If you would like to drink alcohol, don't eat any vegetables or anything else aside from protein. Avoid sweet alcoholic drinks, such as cocktails. The best alcoholic beverages are vodka, tequilla, cognac, and whiskey.

If you are at a restaurant, do not look at the menu, because menus are designed to stimulate your appetite. Decide before you go whether you want to eat animal or plant protein. Ask the server what choices they have, select the one that is consistent with The Happy Body food plan. Most restaurants are happy to provide extra vegetables instead of starches. If you want an alcoholic beverage leave out the vegetables. Follow this guideline until you transition from losing weight to maintenance.

If you are traveling, you will need to take along a sufficient supply of food bars for your snacks, enough to cover you for three bars a day. Be sure to take bars that will not melt in heat. The best choice for this purpose is the original Clif Bar or one of your homemade fruit and nut bars.

If you cross time zones, follow your home schedule on the plane, eating every three hours until you go to sleep at your destination. When you wake up the next day, adapt your schedule to the new time.

There may be occasions when you need to adjust your eating schedule. Some of these occasions may be out of your control, such as getting stuck in traffic or being in a meeting that is running late, and you don't know when you will be able to get back on your regular eating schedule.

The best solution to such emergencies is to always be prepared by having with you at least one of your food bar portions cut into three equal pieces that are wrapped separately. Each piece will cover you for one hour. The following three examples show how to deal with late lunches, but the same kind of adjustments can be made for late dinners.

Example 1: Eating Lunch One Hour Late

If you should have to eat lunch one hour later than usual—say, at 1:00 p.m. instead of 12:00 p.m., you should eat one portion of your bar at 12:00. Then you have your whole lunch at 1:00 and your next snack at 4:00 instead of 3:00. Since it is only two hours to your dinner, you take only two of your three portions at 4:00, and have a full dinner at 6:00 (see Table 7.1).

We have observed with many of our clients who are at the beginning of the program that the people around them will challenge them.

Example 2: Eating Lunch Two Hours Late

If you should have to eat lunch two hours later than usual—say, at 2:00 p.m. instead of 12:00 p.m., you should eat one portion of your bar at 12:00 and another portion at 1:00. Then you have your whole lunch at 2:00 and your next snack at 5:00 instead of 3:00. Since it is only one hour to your normal dinnertime, you take only one of your three portions at 5:00, and have a full dinner at 6:00 (see Table 7.1).

Example 3: Eating Lunch Three Hours Late

If you should have to eat lunch three hours later than usual—say, at 3:00 p.m. instead of 12:00 p.m., you should eat one portion of your bar at 12:00, another portion at 1:00, and a third portion at 2:00. Then you have your whole lunch at 3:00 and your dinner at 6:00 (see Table 7.1).

Very rarely, you may need to eat earlier than usual, for some special reason. An example of this is illustrated in Table 7.2 for Thursday.

TABLE 7.1: ADJUSTING YOUR LUNCH SCHEDULE

Time	1 Hour Later	2 Hours Later	3 Hours Later
6:00 am			
7:00			
8:00			
9:00	Snack	Snack	Snack
10:00			
11:00			
12:00 pm	⅓ of Snack	⅓ of Snack	⅓ of Snack
1:00	Lunch	⅓ of Snack	⅓ of Snack
2:00		Lunch	⅓ of Snack
3:00			Lunch
4:00	⅔ of Snack		
5:00		⅓ of Snack	
6:00	Dinner	Dinner	Dinner
7:00			
8:00			
9:00	Snack	Snack	Snack
10:00			

You should keep a food journal to learn about yourself and your eating habits. It is important to see in writing what your are eating and when.

Keeping Your Food Journal

You should keep a food journal to learn about yourself and your eating habits (see Table 7.2). In the beginning, you will probably make many notes in your daily journal, such as comments about your mood, energy, and pains or discomforts. Indicate how things are getting better or worse. It is very important to see in writing what you are eating and when. This will help to clarify for you exactly what needs to be changed and make it harder for you to fool yourself.

After a month or so, you will probably develop patterns and need to write less (for an example, see Table 7.3). At that point, you can keep a weekly rather than a daily journal, which will help you to observe your weekly patterns (see Table 7.4).

Once you have achieved your Ideal Body Weight and Ideal Body Weight Proportions, you will have developed such strong eating habits that you will probably no longer need to keep a journal.

Banquet Day

Once you have achieved your Ideal Body Weight, you can give yourself an occasional feast for a meal, but not more than once per week. At such times, you can eat as much as you want and whatever you want. Your body does not have the capacity to convert all these calories into fat, so instead it will eliminate most of them. Nevertheless, in only a few hours, you will gain 3 to 4 percent of your total body weight.

A 200-pound man could gain as much as eight pounds. But most of this will be retained water. If you return to your food plan the day after the banquet, your appetite will return to normal within three or four days, and you will lose the pounds you gained.

The only problem with banqueting is that your metabolism goes up and your stomach is stretched, so you will be tempted on the following day to overeat. Knowing that you will face this temptation will make it easier for you to resist it. After three or four days, the craving will disappear, and your weight will have returned to normal.

Some of our clients like to schedule a regular weekly banquet day and have no problem maintaining their Ideal Body Weight. This allows them to go back to their old pleasures once a week without gaining weight. Other clients prefer to avoid banqueting except for very special occasions, such as parties, holiday dinners, and weddings. We have noticed that, over time, most of our clients tend to reduce the size and frequency of their banquets.

A Special Note to Vegetarians

Many of our clients are vegetarians. The only adjustments they have to make in The Happy Body eating program is their choice of protein for lunch and dinner. The volumes by gram and by fist size are the same.

TABLE 7.2: EXAMPLE OF MY WEEKLY FOOD JOURNAL

Week – From: 2-18-08   **To:** 2-24-09

Time	Mon	Tue	Wed	Thu	Fri	Sat	Sun
Morning Weight:	146	145.8	145.5	146.6	145.3	145.3	144.7
6:00 am				banana & cashews			
7:00		men's bread					
8:00			yogurt & orange				
9:00	hemp bread			2/3 larabar	women's bread		
10:00		1/3 builder bar				6 egg-wh. omelet	berries & walnuts
11:00		apple & almonds	2/3 clif bar	organic bar			
12:00 pm	protein burger				yogurt & strawberry		
1:00			1/3 clif bar			yogurt & peach	rice & snow peas
2:00		rice & green bns.	chicken salad	1/3 larabar			
3:00	yogurt & blueberry			sashimi & cucumbers	barley & mushrms		
4:00						soy beans & salsa	hemp bread
5:00		2/3 builder bar	men's bread				
6:00	beans & peppers			chicken & caulifl.	flavor & fiber		
7:00		sea bass & vodka				greens + bar	swordfish & asparag.
8:00			quinoa & salad				
9:00	luna bar				cheese & wine		
10:00						shrimp & beer	think thin bar
Evening Weight:	147.8	147.3	148.7	147.4	146.8	146.5	146.3

TABLE 7.3: MY DAILY FOOD JOURNAL

Date:	Morning Weight:		Evening Weight:
Time	**Food**		**Notes**
6:00 am			
7:00			
8:00			
9:00			
10:00			
11:00			
12:00 pm			
1:00			
2:00)			
3:00			
4:00			
5:00			
6:00			
7:00			
8:00			
9:00			
10:00			

COPY THIS FORM FOR YOUR OWN PERSONAL USE

TABLE 7.4: MY WEEKLY FOOD JOURNAL							
Week – From:		**To:**					
Time	**Mon**	**Tue**	**Wed**	**Thu**	**Fri**	**Sat**	**Sun**
Morning Weight:							
6:00 am							
7:00							
8:00							
9:00							
10:00							
11:00							
12:00 pm							
1:00							
2:00							
3:00							
4:00							
5:00							
6:00							
7:00							
8:00							
9:00							
10:00							
Evening Weight:							

When All Else Fails

Ray Walton (60-year-old real estate agent)

During the past ten years, hoping to lose weight and become healthier, I trained for a marathon but had to drop out after 15 miles due to severe back pain.

Then I spent several months in a boot camp training program, running up and down the stadium bleachers, doing pushups and jogging several miles a day. But my back was still killing me.

To eliminate the pounding action of running, which worsened the back pain, I switched to cycling. Soon I was riding 150 to 200 miles a week to prepare myself for a 500-mile bike ride. But when it was over, I found that I had gained more weight than I had lost, and my back was still hurting.

Next, I joined a weight loss program and lost 25 pounds in a relatively short time but gained back 35 pounds soon after I stopped the program.

In addition to my weight problem and my chronic back pain, my blood pressure was 150/90 *with* medication, and my cholesterol, which had always been low, reached 250.

The pain medication and anti-inflammatory drugs that I had taken for seven years for my back were withdrawn from the market, so I started taking up to two dozen ibuprofen a day simply to manage the pain. I was desperate. Nothing had worked. At 6'1", I weighed 235 pounds — much more than what I had weighed in 1991.

Then, at my company's annual Christmas party, I saw a friend who had gone to boot camp with me. She looked fabulous. When I asked her what she had been doing, she told me that she had been training with Jerzy and Aniela Gregorek for several months and gave me their number. I met with them the next day and started The Happy Body program. Since I knew from Pam's example that the program worked, I decided to put my complete trust in Jerzy and Aniela. For the first six weeks of the program, my knees were so bad and creaky that I couldn't do a simple squat, and when I bent over, I couldn't touch the floor. Now, a year later, I can do 240 squats while holding 60 pounds over my head, and I can touch the floor easily. I've lost a total of 50 pounds, while gaining 15 pounds of muscle. My blood pressure has dropped to 110/60, and my cholesterol is 160.

At first, my doctor argued against my discontinuing endurance exercises, but he couldn't argue with the results. Best of all, I'm no longer in pain and *never* take ibuprofen. My life has truly changed. I realize that it is possible not only to stop the aging process, but to reverse it. At 61, I'm in better shape than I've ever been in my life and look forward to continuing this incredible journey.

I am Happy with Me
Teri Hausman (47-year-old host of Beauty Now)

I had no idea that I had become unhealthy. What's especially ironic is that I host a radio show about health, beauty, and diet.

So what happened? As I turned 40, my weight had begun slowly creeping up. I really didn't see it. I'd look at pictures of me and think, "Oh, that is just a bad angle." I played tennis, did step class, rode bikes, and went hiking, but I realized one day that I was 45-years-old and 30 pounds heavier.

My husband and I went to dinner with some friends one evening. One of them had lost about 15 pounds. His wife told me he was working with a couple that were "trainers to the stars" and had this program called The Happy Body.

"Sounds good," I said. I wanted my body back. They warned me: Jerzy and Aniela are tough — they'll tell you to lose 30 or 40 pounds. I remember thinking, "Well that's you, not me. I'm not that heavy."

I was wrong, and I was about to be seriously challenged. The first day of The Happy Body program is picture day – pictures of me in a little swimsuit. Then, I got on their scale. I had always weighed in at 125 to 130, so when the scale tipped at 164 I thought for sure that it was rigged. That was 20 pounds heavier than the day I delivered my kids! As my friend had predicted, Jerzy said I had a good 35 pounds to lose.

I was shocked and upset, but I said, "Okay, show me how." The plan seemed too good to be true. I could still go out and eat at restaurants with friends, but honestly, doing this regularly has probably made me the slowest loser in the program. But Jerzy says, "If the scale is going in the right direction — down — then it is good." If you lose 1 to 2 pounds per month, that's still 12 to 24 pounds in a year.

My success speaks volumes for their methods: To date I have lost about 25 pounds. I wore my bikini in Cabo on vacation and felt great. Twenty-somethings were complimenting me — the mom of a 20-something!

Now I know why they call it The Happy Body. It is not just a way to lose weight but to be happy with your body and yourself. I am now 47 and can't wait until I'm 50, because I figure I'll be in the best shape of my life.

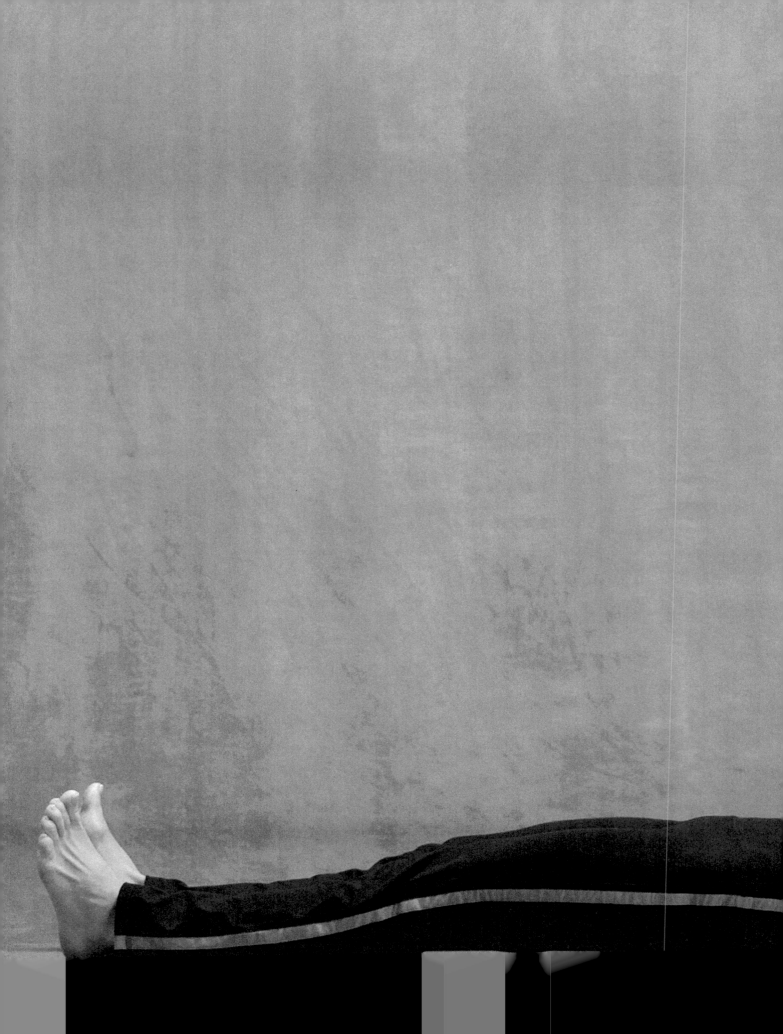

LEARNING
THE
EXERCISES

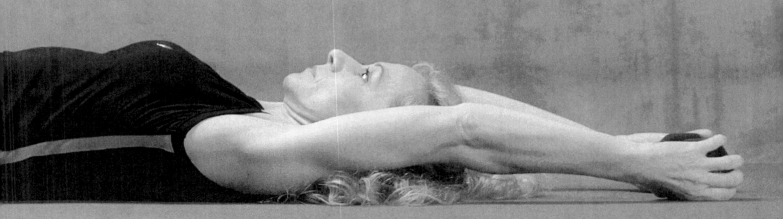

LEARNING A NEW SPORT

L earning The Happy Body program is like learning a new sport. As in swimming, you repeat a limited number of exercises over and over again until you master the techniques. People have various reasons why they choose to learn a sport. Some just want to have fun, others want to win competitions, and still others want to improve their health. All sports are good for your health, but some are better than others. The best ones, because they use the entire body, are the ones we mentioned earlier: baseball, basketball, boxing, figure skating, ice hockey, judo, Olympic weightlifting, Olympic wrestling, pole vaulting, rugby, swimming, volleyball, and water polo. Although these sports help people to improve their health, their principal purpose is competitive, and therefore they frequently lead to injuries as participants push their limits. The Happy Body program, on the other hand, is a noncompetitive sport that is engineered to make your body youthful by mastering eighteen exercises divided into three sequences (1.1–6; 2.1–6; and 3.1–6) and repeating them every day.

WEEK 1 CONTINUED

The Happy Body exercise program promotes a balanced body. Each of the parts of the human body must be in proportion to all the other parts. If any part is out of proportion to the others, injury will result. The shoulder muscles should be stronger than the tricep muscles, which in turn should be stronger than the bicep muscles. If this order of strength is not maintained, problems will follow. For example, if the tricep muscles are stronger than the shoulder muscles, the rotator cuff will not be able to support lifting weight. This could happen when individuals do tricep extensions with more weight than they use when doing shoulder presses.

In The Happy Body program, the weights to be lifted in each of the 18 exercises have been calculated as a percentage of the weight you lift in Exercise 1.1. For example, if you lift 10 pounds in Exercise 1.1, you will lift 50% of that (5 pounds) in Exercises 2.1 and 3.4.

The exercises are designed to measure your progress, no matter what level you begin at. The program will gradually help you to achieve all the Standards of Youthfulness, while at the same time healing any injuries, chronic pains, or other problems you have developed over the years.

Women usually start the program by lifting 3-pound weights in Exercise 1.1 and men by lifting 5-pound weights. Based on your comfort level, you may begin with 1 or 2 more or fewer pounds than this. For Exercises 1.4 through 1.6, follow the percentages given in Table 8.1.

For example, if you determine that you are comfortable lifting 2 pounds in each hand for Exercise 1.1, then, following Table 8.1, you will lift 3 pounds for Exercises 1.4 and 1.6, and 4 pounds for Exercise 1.5.

If, after establishing a comfortable weight for Exercise 1.1, you have trouble with the weight in any of the other three lifting exercises, you need to lower the weight for that exercise until it feels comfortable to raise that weight to the level of the others. Always follow the percentages given for every exercise, even if any of the exercises seem too easy, because that will only prove that your body is out of balance.

Exercises 1, 4, 5, and 6 in all three sequences involve lifting, and Exercises 2 and 3 do not.

Exercises 2 and 3 will always be repeated six times, whereas the number of repetitions for the other four exercises will depend on whether you need to gain muscle (6 repetitions), lose muscle (3 repetitions), or stay the same (3 repetitions).

Always follow the order of exercises in a sequence. When you have completed Sequence 1, start over again from the beginning, and repeat this process six times every day.

In this chapter you will find a break down for all 18 exercises. They have been labeled by Sequence (1,2 & 3) and Exercise (1 - 6) and expressed as Sequence: Exercise (1:1) for the rest of the book.

PERFORM 6 SETS OF 6 REPETITIONS OF EVERY EXERCISE

TABLE 8.1: PERCENTAGES OF WEIGHT LIFTED IN SEQUENCE 1						
SEQUENCE	EXERCISES*					
1	1 100%	2 na	3 na	4 150%	5 200%	6 150%

*If you are not ready for weights, you should perform these exercises without weights.

SEQUENCE	EXERCISE	Standing Tall
1	1	

Description

Into the Exercise (positive lift)

Step 1: Take a dumbbell in each hand, and stand upright with your feet directly under your hips with arms hanging straight down at your sides. Lift your chest, take a deep breath, then curl up your toes and tighten your abdominal and buttocks muscles.

Step 2: While holding your breath, lift your hands to shoulder level without moving your elbows backward. Then continue to Step 3 without pausing.

Step 3: Raise your arms high above your head, keeping your hands a shoulder width apart and the dumbbells parallel to each other throughout the motion until you lock your elbows.

Step 4: Pause and then shift your weight back onto your heels, simultaneously stretching your arms toward the ceiling and slightly tipping your wrists backward so that the dumbbells are higher in the front than in the back. Hold your balance for two seconds.

Out of the Exercise (negative lift):

Step 5: In one continuous movement, release the stretch, return your feet to their normal standing position, lower your arms to the starting position without moving your elbows backward, and exhale as you uncurl your toes and release the tension in your abdominal and buttocks muscles.

Timing & Repetition

The total movement should take at least 11 seconds: 2 seconds for the inhale; 1 second for the positive lift; 1 second for the pause; 1 second for the stretch; 2 seconds for the hold; 2 seconds for the negative lift; and 2 seconds for the exhale. Repeat the exercise 6 times, which should take at least 66 seconds.

Purpose

This exercise has three purposes. First, it will strengthen your shoulders by your lifting heavier weights over time. Second, it will improve the posture of your upper body by enhancing the flexibility of the shoulder blades and decompressing the thoracic spine and rib cage. Third, it will improve your balance by shifting your weight totally onto your heels.

Levels of Difficulty

Level 1: Perform steps 1, 2, and 5.

Level 2: Perform step 1, 2, and 3b (lifting your hands to eye level instead of high above your head), and then perform step 5.

Level 3: Perform steps 1, 2, and 3a (lifting your hands slightly instead of high above your head), and then perform step 5.

Level 4: Perform steps 1, 2, 3, and 5.

Level 5: Perform steps 1–5.

FIGURE 8.1: STANDING TALL

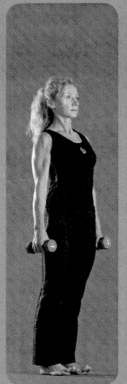
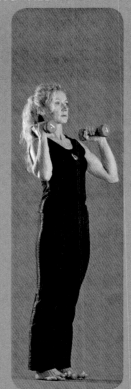
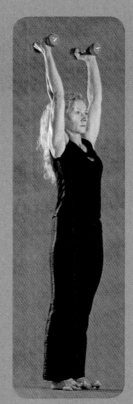
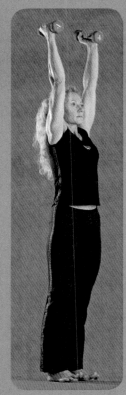
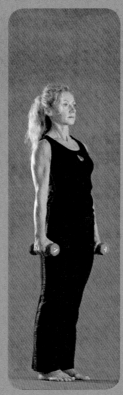

STEP 1   STEP 2   STEP 3   STEP 4   STEP 5

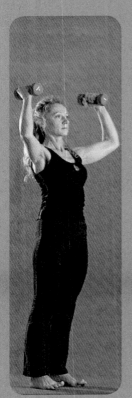
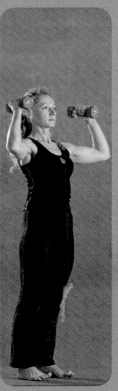

STEP 3a   STEP 3b

SEQUENCE	EXERCISE	
1	2	Cresting Wave

Description

Into the Exercise (positive lift)

Step 1: Lie flat on your back with your arms stretched out above your head and your legs straight up in the air, take a deep breath, then curl your toes toward your face and tighten your abdominal muscles.

Step 2: Raise your arms and head till you touch your toes, and pause.

Step 3: Stretch your arms another inch past your toes as you further tighten your lower abdominal muscles.

Out of the Exercise (negative lift)

Step 4: In one continuous movement, release the stretch, lower your head and arms to their original position, and exhale as you uncurl your toes and release the tension in your abdominal muscles.

Timing & Repetition

The total movement should take at least 9 seconds: 2 seconds for the inhale; 1 second for raising the body; 1 second for the pause; 1 second for the stretch; 1 second for the hold; 1 second for lowering the body; and 2 seconds for the exhale and release. Repeat the exercise 6 times, which should take at least 54 seconds.

Purpose

This exercise has two purposes. First, it will strengthen your abdominal muscles. Second, it will enhance the flexibility of your back.

Levels of Difficulty

Level 1: Perform step 1a, lying flat on your back with your hands behind your head and your legs crossed in the air. Perform step 1b, taking a deep breath and raising your head and shoulders off the floor. Return to the position in step 1a.

Level 2: Perform steps 1 and 2b. Looking straight up, raise your head and shoulders off the floor and point your fingers toward the ceiling. Then perform step 4.

Level 3: Perform steps 1 and 2a. Looking at your toes, take a deep breath and raise your arms and head till your thumbs touch your mid-calves. Then perform step 4.

Level 4: Perform steps 1, 2, and 4.

Level 5: Perform steps 1–4.

FIGURE 8.2: CRESTING WAVE

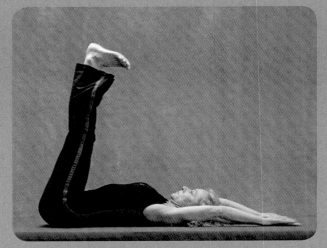

STEP 1

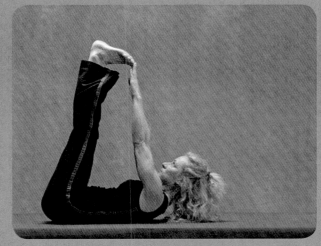

STEP 2

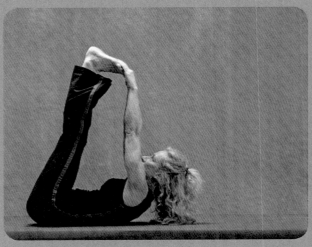

STEP 3

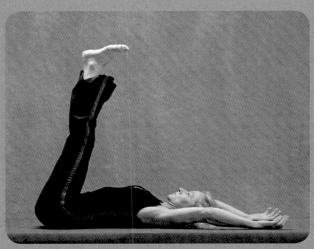

STEP 4

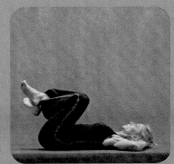

STEP 1a

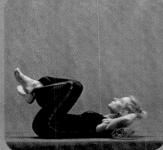

STEP 1b

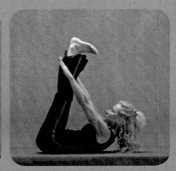

STEP 2a

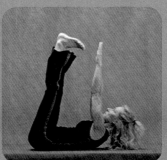

STEP 2b

SEQUENCE 1   EXERCISE 3   Take Off

Description

Into the Exercise (positive lift)

Step 1: Lie on your belly with your arms at your side, your palms facing up, and your head facing to one side. Inhale deeply, then tighten your abdominal, buttocks, and hamstring muscles.

Step 2: Keeping your arms relaxed and your hands and feet touching the floor, raise your upper body, turning your face downward as you do so. Pause for one second.

Step 3: Raise your upper body another inch or two by lifting slightly more off the floor at the waist.

Out of the Exercise (negative lift)

Step 4: In one continuous movement, lower your upper body to the floor, turning your head toward the opposite direction, and then exhale as you relax your abdominal, buttocks, and hamstring muscles.

Timing & Repetition

The total movement should take at least 8 seconds: 2 seconds for the inhale; 1 second for raising the body; 1 second for the pause; 1 second for the extension; 1 second for lowering the body; and 2 seconds for the exhale and release. Repeat the exercise 6 times, which should take at least 48 seconds.

Purpose

This exercise has three purposes. First, it will strengthen your lumbar muscles. Second, it will enhance the flexibility of your back. Third, it will enhance your neck's range of motion by stretching your trapezius, sternocleidomastoid, rib cage, and related muscles.

Levels of Difficulty

Level 1: Perform step 1a, which is identical to step 1 except with your with your elbows bent upward at 90 degrees. Perform step 1b, using your arms to raise your upper body so that your nose is a few inches from the floor. Then, turning your head in the opposite direction, return to your position in step 1a.

Level 2: Perform steps 1 and 2b. Keeping your arms relaxed and your hands and feet touching the floor, raise your upper body about a quarter as much as in step 2. Then perform step 4.

Level 3: Perform steps 1 and 2a. Keeping your arms relaxed and your hands and feet touching the floor, raise your upper body about half as much as in step 2. Then perform step 4.

Level 4: Perform steps 1, 2, and 4.

Level 5: Perform steps 1–4.

FIGURE 8.3: TAKE OFF

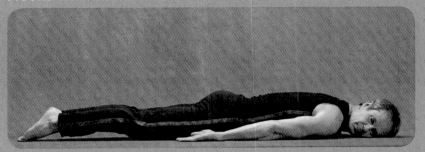

STEP 1

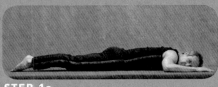

STEP 1a

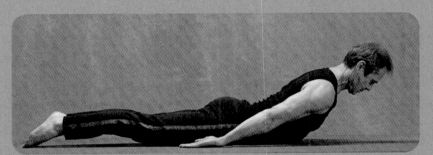

STEP 2

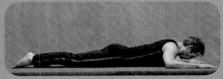

STEP 1b

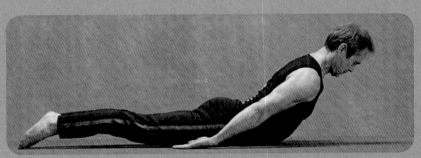

STEP 3

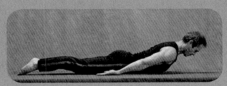

STEP 2a

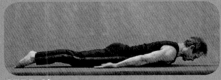

STEP 2b

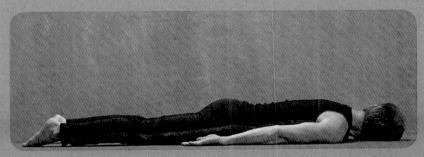

STEP 4

Tapping Hammer

Description

Into the Exercise (positive lift)

Step 1: Take a dumbbell in both hands and raise it over and behind your head, with the lower end of the dumbbell at shoulder height, holding it between your thumbs. Lift your chest, take a deep breath, and then curl up your toes and tighten your abdominal and buttocks muscles.

Step 2: While holding your breath, lift your hands straight up, lock your elbows, and pause.

Step 3: Shift your weight back onto your heels, simultaneously stretching your arms further toward the ceiling. Hold your balance for two seconds.

Out of the Exercise (negative lift):

Step 4: In one continuous motion, release the stretch, return your feet to their normal position, lower your hands to the starting position, and exhale as you uncurl your toes and release the tension in your abdominal and buttocks muscles.

Timing & Repetition

The total movement should take at least 11 seconds: 2 seconds for the inhale; 1 second for the positive lift; 1 second for the pause; 1 second for the stretch; 2 seconds for the hold; 2 seconds for the negative lift; and 2 seconds for the exhale and release. Repeat the exercise 6 times, which should take at least 66 seconds.

Purpose

This exercise has four purposes. First, it will strengthen your tricep muscles. Second, it will improve the posture of your upper body by enhancing the flexibility of the shoulder blades and decompressing the thoracic spine and rib cage. Third, it will improve your balance by shifting your weight totally onto your heels. Fourth, it will improve the flexibility of your wrists.

Levels of Difficulty

Level 1: Holding the dumbbell horizontally, but lying on your back, perform step 1a (inhale deeply, then tighten your abdominal and buttock muscles and rotate your ankles and curl your toes toward your face). Perform step 1b (lift the dumbbell until your arms are pointed straight up). Perform step 1c (stretch your arms further toward the ceiling). Perform step 1d (in one continuous motion, lower your hands to the starting position and exhale as you uncurl your toes, unrotate your ankles, and release the tension in your abdominal and buttock muscles).

Level 2: Holding the dumbbell horizontally, perform steps 1, 2, and 4.

Level 3: Holding the dumbbell vertically, perform steps 1, 2, and 4.

Level 4: Holding the dumbbell horizontally instead of vertically, perform steps 1–4.

Level 5: Perform steps 1–4.

FIGURE 8.4: TAPPING HAMMER

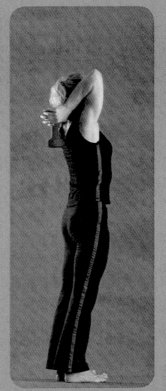

STEP 1

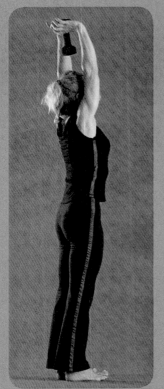

STEP 2

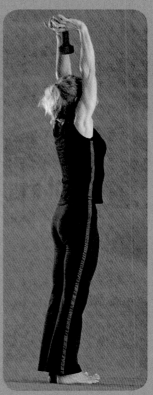

STEP 3

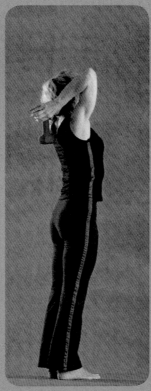

STEP 4

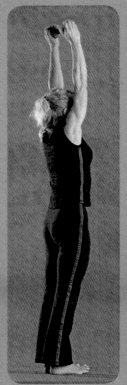

**HOLDING THE
DUMBBELL
HORIZONTALLY**

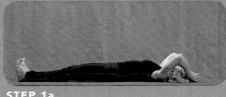

STEP 1a

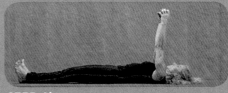

STEP 1b

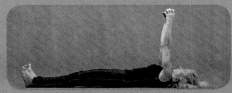

STEP 1c

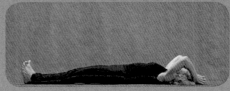

STEP 1d

SEQUENCE	EXERCISE	
1	**5**	**Sitting Tower**

Description

Into the Exercise (positive lift)

Step 1: Stand with your feet a shoulder length apart and your toes pointed outward. Hold a dumbbell under your chin, resting on your shoulders, with your elbows pointed forward. Lift your chest, take a deep breath, then flex your abdominal muscles and curl your toes upward.

Step 2: While holding your breath, lower yourself into a squat position without bending forward or lowering your elbows or raising your heels. Then immediately stand up straight.

Out of the Exercise (negative lift):

Step 3: Exhale as you uncurl your toes and release the tension in your abdominal muscles.

Timing & Repetition

The total movement should take at least 6 seconds: 2 seconds for the inhale; 2 seconds for the squat; and 2 seconds for the exhale and release. Repeat the exercise 6 times, which should take at least 36 seconds.

Purpose

This exercise has three purposes. First, it will strengthen your thigh, buttocks, and lower back muscles. Second, it will improve the flexibility of your ankles, knees, hips, spine, shoulders, triceps, trapezius, and wrists. Third, it will enhance your posture and balance by forcing your spine to arch backward throughout the exercise.

Levels of Difficulty

Level 1: Perform steps 1, 2d (squatting slightly), and 3.

Level 2: Perform steps 1, 2c, and 3, using a low table or bench.

Level 3: Perform steps 1, 2b, and 3, using a low table or bench.

Level 4: Perform steps 1, 2a, and 3, using a low table or bench.

Level 5: Perform steps 1–3.

FIGURE 8.5: SITTING TOWER

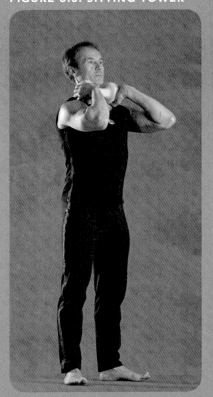

STEP 1

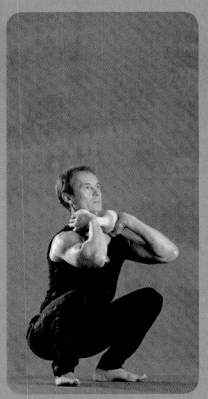

STEP 2

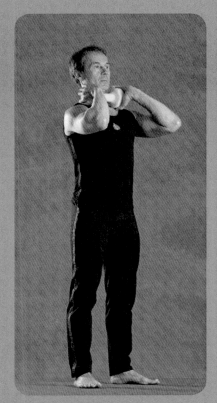

STEP 3

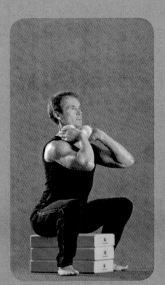

STEP 2a

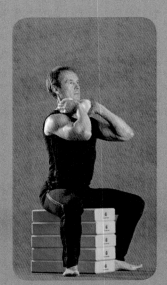

STEP 2b

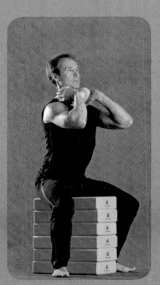

STEP 2c

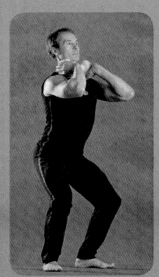

STEP 2d

SEQUENCE **1** EXERCISE **6** Take a Bow

Description

Into the Exercise (positive lift)

Step 1: Take a dumbbell in each hand and stand upright with your feet wide apart, your toes facing outward 45 degrees, and your arms hanging straight down in front of you. Lift your chest and take a deep breath, then curl up your toes, lock your knees, and tighten your abdominal muscles.

Step 2: While holding your breath and keeping your knees locked, bend forward till the dumbbells touch the ground.

Step 3: Without pausing, stand up straight and tighten your buttocks muscles.

Step 4: Stand on your toes and simultaneously lift your shoulders to your ears, holding this pose for two seconds.

Out of the Exercise (negative lift):

Step 5: In one continuous movement, release the stretch, return your feet to the starting position, and exhale as you release the tension in your abdominal and buttocks muscles.

Timing & Repetition

The total movement should take at least 10 seconds: 2 seconds for the inhale; 1 second for bending forward; 1 second for the lift; 1 second for the stretch; 2 seconds for the hold; 1 second for lowering your shoulders and heels; and 2 seconds for the exhale and release. Repeat the exercise 6 times, which should take at least 60 seconds.

Purpose

This exercise has three purposes. First, it will strengthen your hamstrings and lower back. Second, it will improve the flexibility of your trapezium muscles, spine, hamstrings, and calves. Third, it will improve your balance by shifting your weight totally onto your toes.

Levels of Difficulty

Level 1: Perform steps 1, 2d (mid-thigh level), 3, 4, and 5.

Level 2: Perform steps 1, 2c (knee level), 3, 4, and 5.

Level 3: Perform steps 1, 2b (mid-shin level), 3, 4, and 5.

Level 4: Perform steps 1, 2a (ankle level), 3, 4, and 5.

Level 5: Perform steps 1–5.

SEQUENCE 1, EXERCISE 6

FIGURE 8.6: TAKE A BOW

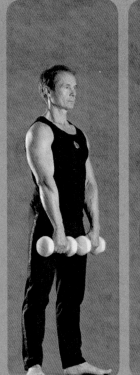
STEP 1

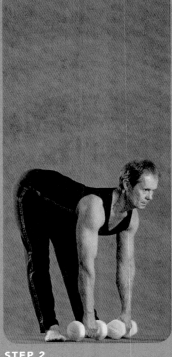
STEP 2

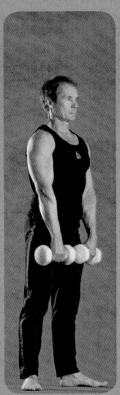
STEP 3

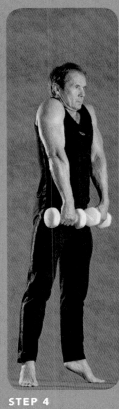
STEP 4

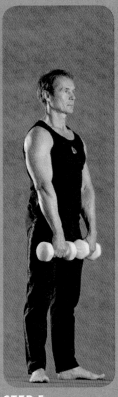
STEP 5

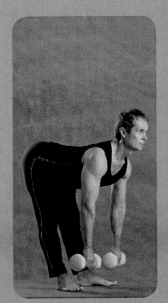
STEP 2a

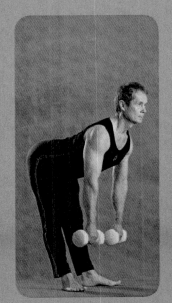
STEP 2b

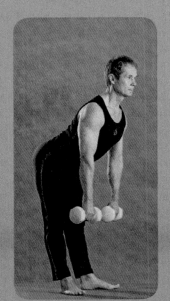
STEP 2c

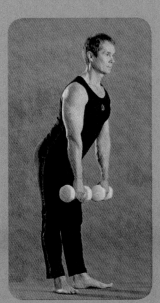
STEP 2d

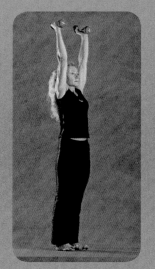

**SEQUENCE 1
EXERCISE 1**

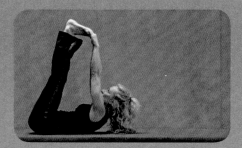

**SEQUENCE 1
EXERCISE 2**

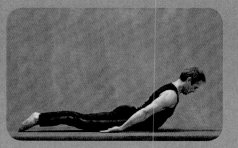

**SEQUENCE 1
EXERCISE 3**

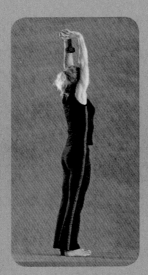

**SEQUENCE 1
EXERCISE 4**

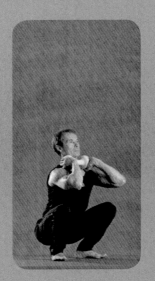

**SEQUENCE 1
EXERCISE 5**

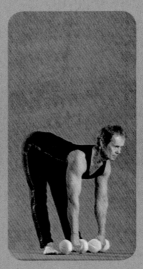

**SEQUENCE 1
EXERCISE 6**

My Own True Fairy Tale

Gwen Fuller (50-year-old life coach)

Once upon a time, there was a girl name Gwen, whose life was transformed when she witnessed Peggy Fleming win the gold medal in figure skating in the 1968 Olympics. "Someday, I too will skate inspiring performances for arenas full of people," she proclaimed. At first, everyone said, "That's nice." Before long, however, she was skating 6 hours a day. She had never felt so exhilarated as when she was skating as fast as she could, spinning and jumping, almost defying gravity. Gwen's body was very happy.

When she grew up, Gwen shifted her life's focus to raising a family and becoming a life coach, but she made sure to rollerblade almost every day so she could still feel the thrill of the wind on her face as she sped along. Everything seemed wonderful—she looked athletic and fulfilled at age 40. But this was an illusion. Her body was in trouble. As part of a "wellness" check-up, she took a bone-density scan that revealed osteoporosis. She was devastated—her bones were as porous and brittle as those of an average 85-year-old woman! Gwen's body was miserable.

So, at age 40 (85…), she went to the very best doctors, who all gave her the same dire warning, "You will shatter if you fall, so it's urgent that you rebuild your bones." Her beloved skating was forbidden. In fact, almost any physical activity might be dangerous. Gwen was already taking calcium supplements, and she seemed like she was in great shape, so what more could she do? Five years passed as she consulted with physical therapists, personal trainers, and elite training centers, but none offered any legitimate and comprehensive, successful formula for improving bone quality. Gwen's body was in limbo.

As a life coach, Gwen refused to abandon hope, and used her frustration, fear, and anger to fuel her quest to find a daily routine that would rehabilitate her body. Finally, at age 48, she happened upon an article about the Gregoreks and The Happy Body program. She was so impressed by their philosophy, technique, and knowledge of physiology, that she boldly tracked down Jerzy's number and called his cell phone. He answered, and Gwen's body was on the road to recovery.

Nearly two years have passed and Gwen has consistently practiced The Happy Body workout that Jerzy and Aniela designed specifically for her. When her recent bone-density scan showed her bones to be above average for her age, the doctor who read the results, called them "heroic." Additionally, The Happy Body workout has improved Gwen's posture, flexibility, and strength. She has been given the green light to skate to her heart's content. Thanks to Jerzy and Aniela, at age 50 Gwen's body is truly happy once again.

WEEK 2

Reviewing Your Food Program

By now, after one week, depending on your body type, you should have lost or gained 1% of your Ideal Body Weight.

If you have lost more than 1% of your Ideal Body Weight, you were probably allergic to some of the foods you used to eat, and therefore your body was inflamed and bloated—that is, you were carrying excess water. On the other hand, if you have lost less than 1% of your Ideal Body Weight, which is extremely rare, you must either not be eating on the three-hour schedule or you have a low metabolism rate and must eat even less than you are eating now. In the latter case, try lowering your snack intake by 10%.

If you have gained more than 1% of your Ideal Body Weight, your body was probably deprived of nutrients, and now your muscles are absorbing more water. On the other hand, if you have gained less than 1% of your Ideal Body Weight, you either are not eating enough or are not exercising regularly.

Reviewing Your Exercise Program

If, after performing Sequence 1 of the exercises for a week, your body or any part of it is sore or stiff, repeat Sequence 1 of the exercises for the following week, but go down one level of difficulty in whatever exercises seem to be causing the problem. If you go all the way down to Level 1 and the problem persists, reduce the weight of your dumbbells by one pound until the problem ceases.

If your body or any part of it is not sore or stiff, and if the dumbbells you are lifting feel comfortable, learn Sequence 2 and perform it every day after you complete Sequence 1. In this case, however, instead of repeating the sequences six times, repeat each of them four times.

For Exercises 2.1 through 2.6, follow the percentages given in Table 8.2.

For example, if you determined that you were comfortable lifting 2 pounds for Exercise 1.1, then, following Table 8.2, you will lift 1 pound for Exercise 2.1, 4 pounds for Exercise 2.4, 2 pounds for Exercise 2.5, and 3 pounds for Exercise 2.6.

PERFORM 4 SETS OF 6 REPETITIONS OF EVERY EXERCISE

TABLE 8.2: PERCENTAGES OF WEIGHT LIFTED IN SEQUENCES 1 AND 2						
SEQUENCE	EXERCISES					
1	1 100%	2 na	3 na	4 150%	5 200%	6 150%
2	1 50%	2 na	3 na	4 200%	5 100%	6 150%

SEQUENCE | EXERCISE
2 1 Opening Wide

Description

Into the Exercise (positive lift)

Step 1: Place two dumbbells on the floor, parallel to each other, the distance of your outstretched arms. Lie down between them so that they are at shoulder level, and take one in each hand. Inhale deeply, then tighten your abdominal and buttocks muscles as you rotate your ankles and curl your toes toward your face.

Step 2: While holding your breath, lock your elbows and lift your arms straight up until they are a shoulder width apart.

Step 3: Pause and then stretch your arms further toward the ceiling.

Out of the Exercise (negative lift):

Step 4: In one continuous movement, release the stretch, return your arms to the floor, uncurl your toes, unrotate your ankles, and exhale as you release the tension in your abdominal and buttocks muscles.

Timing & Repetition

The total movement should take at least 10 seconds: 2 seconds for the inhale; 1 second for the positive lift; 1 second for the pause; 1 second for the stretch; 1 second for the hold; 2 seconds for the negative lift; and 2 seconds for the exhale and release. Repeat the exercise 6 times, which should take at least 60 seconds.

Purpose

This exercise has two purposes. First, it will strengthen your front deltoid and pectoral muscles. Second, it will enhance the flexibility of your front deltoid, pectoral, and bicep muscles.

Levels of Difficulty

Level 1: Perform step 1a (lie on the floor with the dumbbells at your hips, then rotate the dumbbells so that they are standing on the floor; inhale deeply, then tighten your abdominal and buttock muscles as you rotate your ankles and curl your toes toward your face).

Perform step 1b (bend your elbows 90 degrees).

Perform step 1c (while holding your breath, lift your arms straight up until they are locked and a shoulder width apart).

Perform step 1e (releasing the stretch), 1f (lowering your elbows to the floor), and 1g (exhaling and releasing tension).

Level 2: Perform step 1a, 1b, 1c. Perform step 1d (stretch your arms further toward the ceiling).

Perform step 1e (releasing the stretch), 1f, and 1g.

Level 3: Without locking your elbows, perform steps 1, 2, and 4.

Level 4: Perform steps 1, 2, and 4.

Level 5: Perform steps 1–4.

FIGURE 8.7: OPENING WIDE

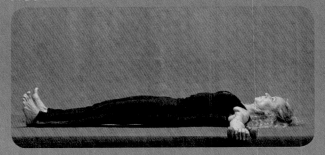

STEP 1

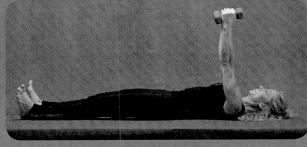

STEP 2

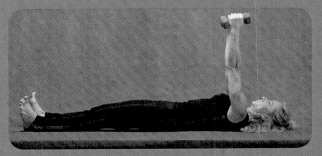

STEP 3

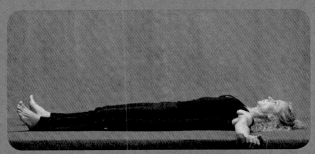

STEP 4

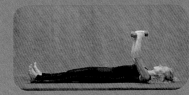

UNLOCKED ELBOWS
(LEVEL 3)

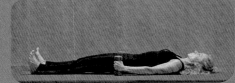

STEP 1a

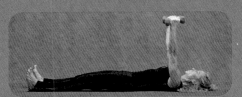

STEP 1e

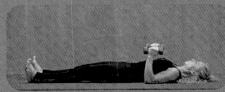

STEP 1b

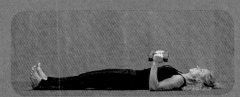

STEP 1f

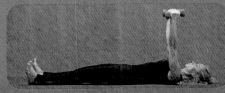

STEP 1c

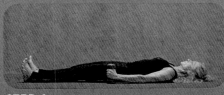

STEP 1g

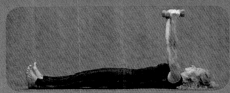

STEP 1d

SEQUENCE	EXERCISE	
2	2	Shifting Wave

Description

Into the Exercise (positive lift)

Step 1: Lie flat on your back with your arms stretched out above your head and your legs straight up in the air. Rotate your ankles and curl your toes toward your face.

Step 2: Looking at your toes, take a deep breath, and, while placing one arm alongside your body with your palm extended, raise your head and other arm till you touch the toes of your opposite foot, and pause.

Step 3: Tighten your abdominal muscles and stretch both arms another inch or two.

Out of the Exercise (negative lift)

Step 4: Release the stretch, lower your head and arms to their original position, and exhale as you uncurl your toes, unrotate your ankles, and release the tension in your abdominal muscles.

Timing & Repetition

The total movement should take at least 9 seconds: 2 seconds for the inhale; 1 second for raising the body; 1 second for the pause; 1 second for the stretch; 1 second for the hold; 1 second for lowering the body; and 2 seconds for the exhale and release. Repeat the exercise 6 times, alternating sides, which should take at least 54 seconds.

Purpose

This exercise has two purposes. First, it will strengthen your oblique muscles. Second, it will enhance the flexibility of your back.

Levels of Difficulty

Level 1: Lie flat on your back with your hands behind your head and your legs crossed in the air (step 1a). Take a deep breath, then tighten your abdominal muscles. Raise your head and one shoulder off the floor so that your elbow points toward the ceiling (step 1b). Return to the original position and exhale as you release the tension in your abdominal muscles.

Level 2: Perform steps 1 and 2b (pointing your arm straight up). Then perform step 4.

Level 3: Perform steps 1 and 2a (touching your palm to the outside of the calf of the opposite leg). Then perform step 4.

Level 4: Perform steps 1, 2, and 4.

Level 5: Perform steps 1–4.

FIGURE 8.8: SHIFTING WAVE

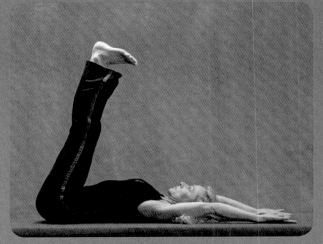

STEP 1

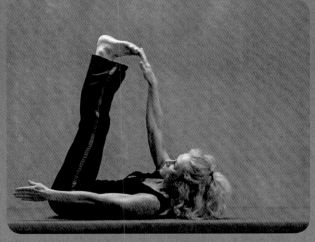

STEP 2

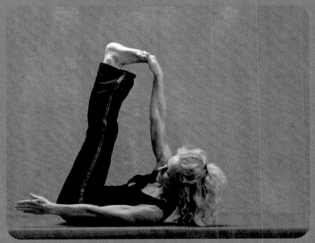

STEP 3

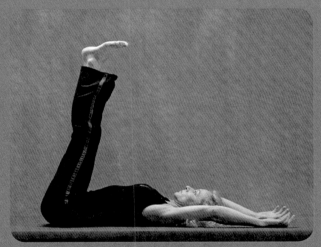

STEP 4

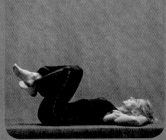

STEP 1a

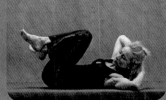

STEP 1b

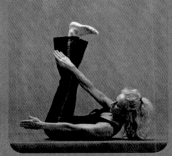

STEP 2a

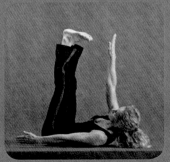

STEP 2b

SEQUENCE 2 — EXERCISE 3 — Fly Up

Description

Into the Exercise (positive lift)

Step 1: Lie on your belly with your head facing to one side. Place your hands just above your head. Inhale deeply.

Step 2: Keeping your elbows touching the floor, raise your upper body so that you are looking straight ahead. Pause for one second.

Step 3: Looking up toward the ceiling, raise your head another inch or two.

Out of the Exercise (negative lift)

Step 4: Lower your head to the floor, facing toward the opposite direction. Exhale and release.

Timing & Repetition

The total movement should take at least 8 seconds: 2 seconds for the inhale; 1 second for raising the body; 1 second for the pause; 1 second for the extension; 1 second for lowering the body; and 2 seconds for the exhale and release. Repeat the exercise 6 times, which should take at least 48 seconds.

Purpose

This exercise has three purposes. First, it will strengthen your upper back muscles. Second, it will enhance the flexibility of your rib cage. Third, it will enhance your neck's range of motion by stretching your trapezius, sternocleidomastoid, and related muscles.

Levels of Difficulty

Level 1: Perform steps 1, 2c (looking down at the floor), and 4.

Level 2: Perform steps 1, 2b (looking at your fingertips), and 4.

Level 3: Perform steps 1, 2a (looking in front of your fingertips), and 4.

Level 4: Perform steps 1, 2, and 4.

Level 5: Perform steps 1–4.

FIGURE 8.9: FLY UP

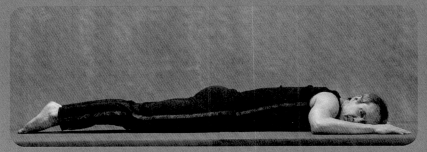

STEP 1

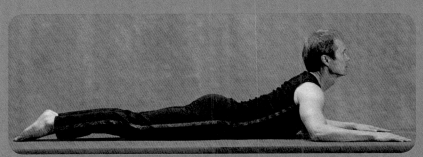

STEP 2

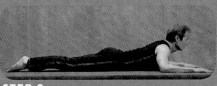

STEP 2a

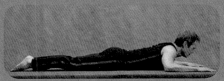

STEP 2b

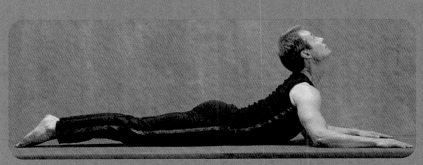

STEP 3

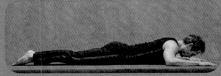

STEP 2c

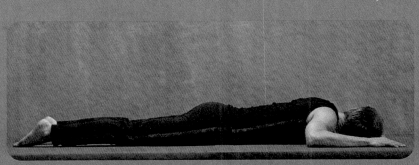

STEP 4

SEQUENCE **2** EXERCISE **4** Rocking Trunk

Description

Into the Exercise (positive lift)

Step 1: Stand with your legs a shoulder width apart, with a dumbbell lying on the floor between your feet. Bend forward so that your back is parallel to the ground, place one hand on the same-side knee, and twist your torso so that you can place your other hand on the dumbbell. Inhale deeply, then flex your abdominal muscles and curl your toes upward.

Step 2: While holding your breath, lift the dumbbell by raising your arm and untwisting your torso until the back of the dumbbell is level with your upper thigh.

Step 3: Pause and then, keeping your arm in the same position relative to your torso, twist your torso upward another two or three inches.

Out of the Exercise (negative lift)

Step 4: In one continuous movement, release the stretch, return the dumbbell to the floor so that you are now back in the starting position, and exhale as you uncurl your toes and release the tension in your abdominal muscles.

Timing & Repetition

The total movement should take at least 9 seconds: 2 seconds for the inhale; 1 second for the lift; 1 second for the pause; 1 second for the twist; 2 seconds for returning to the original position; and 2 seconds for the exhale and release. Repeat the exercise 6 times for each arm, which should take at least 54 seconds each.

Purpose

This exercise has two purposes. First, it will strengthen your deltoid muscles and your latissimus dorsi muscles (i.e., your middle back muscles, commonly called "lats"). Second, it will enhance the flexibility of your rib cage.

Levels of Difficulty

Level 1: Perform steps 1b–4, but with one hand resting on a surface that is at knee level and the dumbbell at mid-calf level.

Level 2: Perform steps 1a, 2, and 4, but with one hand resting on a surface that is at mid-calf level.

Level 3: Perform steps 1a–4, but with one hand resting on a surface that is at mid-calf level.

Level 4: Perform steps 1, 2, and 4.

Level 5: Perform steps 1–4.

FIGURE 8.10: ROCKING TRUNK

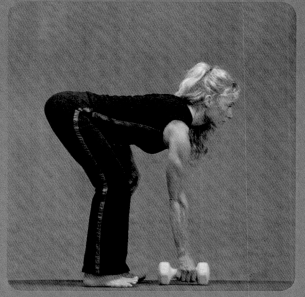

STEP 1

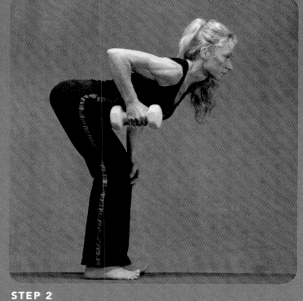

STEP 2

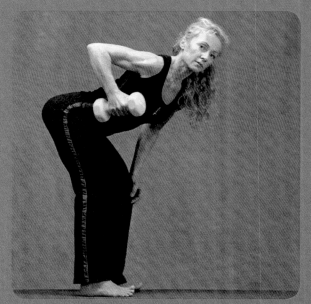

STEP 3

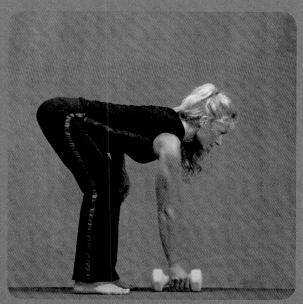

STEP 4

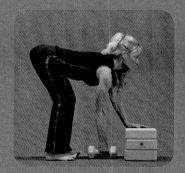

STEP 1a

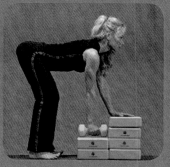

STEP 1b

Rising Tower

Description

Into the Exercise (positive lift)

Step 1: Holding dumbbells at your sides, stand with your feet a shoulder width apart and your toes pointed outward. Lift your chest and inhale deeply, then flex your abdominal muscles and curl your toes upward.

Steps 2, 3, & 4: In a continuous movement, without moving your elbows backward, lift the dumbbells parallel to each other until they are at chin level, then rotate your arms backward.

Steps 5, 6, & 7: Press the dumbbells above your head until your elbows lock. Squat without bending forward or raising your heels, and immediately stand up straight.

Out of the Exercise (negative lift):

Steps 8, 9, 10, & 11: In a continuous movement, lower the dumbbells to chin level; rotate your arms forward, and lower the dumbbells in front of you to the starting position without moving your elbows backward. Then exhale as you uncurl your toes and release the tension in your abdominal muscles.

Timing & Repetition

The total movement should take at least 9 seconds: 2 seconds for the inhale; 1 second for the press; 2 seconds for the squat; 2 seconds for lowering the dumbbells; and 2 seconds for the exhale and release. Repeat the exercise 6 times, which should take at least 54 seconds.

Purpose

This exercise has three purposes. First, it will strengthen your thigh, buttock, lower back, and deltoid muscles. Second, it will improve the flexibility of your ankles, knees, hips, spine, shoulders, and wrists. Third, it will enhance your posture and balance by forcing your spine to arch backward throughout the exercise.

Levels of Difficulty

Level 1: Perform steps 1–5, 6d (squatting slightly), 7–11.

Level 2: Using a low table or bench, perform steps 1–5, 6c, 7–11.

Level 3: Using a low table or bench, perform steps 1–5, 6b, 7–11.

Level 4: Using a low table or bench, perform steps 1–5, 6a, 7–11.

Level 5: Perform steps 1–11.

FIGURE 8.11: RISING TOWER

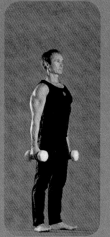 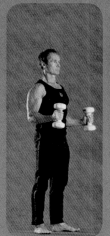 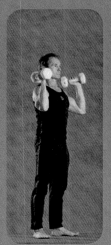 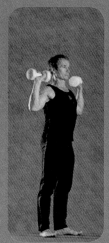 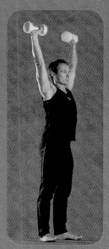 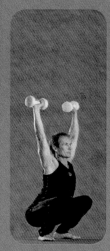

STEP 1   STEP 2   STEP 3   STEP 4   STEP 5   STEP 6

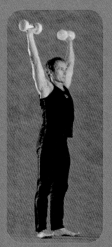 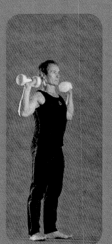 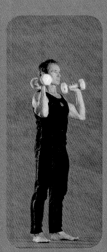 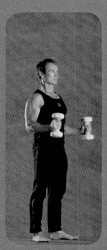 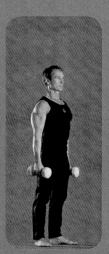

STEP 7   STEP 8   STEP 9   STEP 10   STEP 11

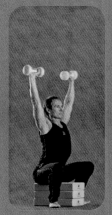 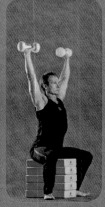 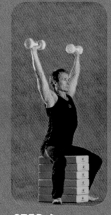 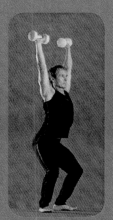

STEP 6a   STEP 6b   STEP 6c   STEP 6d

SEQUENCE 2 EXERCISE 6 Encore Bow

Description

Into the Exercise (positive lift)

Step 1: Take a dumbbell in each hand, and stand upright with your feet directly under your hips with arms hanging straight down at your sides. Lift your chest and take a deep breath, then curl up your toes, lock your knees, and tighten your abdominal muscles.

Step 2: While holding your breath and keeping your knees locked, bend forward till the dumbbells touch the ground.

Step 3: Without pausing, stand up straight and tighten your buttocks muscles.

Step 4: Stand on your toes and simultaneously lift your shoulders to your ears, holding this pose for two seconds.

Out of the Exercise (negative lift):

Step 5: In one continuous movement, release the stretch, return your feet to the starting position, and exhale as you release the tension in your abdominal and buttocks muscles.

Timing & Repetition

The total movement should take at least 10 seconds: 2 seconds for the inhale; 1 second for bending forward; 1 second for the lift; 1 second for the stretch; 2 seconds for the hold; 1 second for lowering your shoulders and heels, and 2 seconds for the exhale and release. Repeat the exercise 6 times, which should take at least 60 seconds.

Purpose

This exercise has three purposes. First, it will strengthen your hamstrings and lower back. Second, it will improve the flexibility of your trapezium muscles, spine, hamstrings, and calves. Third, it will improve your balance by shifting your weight totally onto your toes.

Levels of Difficulty

Level 1: Perform steps 1, 2d (mid-thigh level), 3, 4, and 5.

Level 2: Perform steps 1, 2c (knee level), 3, 4, and 5.

Level 3: Perform steps 1, 2b (mid-shin level), 3, 4, and 5.

Level 4: Perform steps 1, 2a (ankle level), 3, 4, and 5.

Level 5: Perform steps 1–5.

FIGURE 8.12: ENCORE BOW

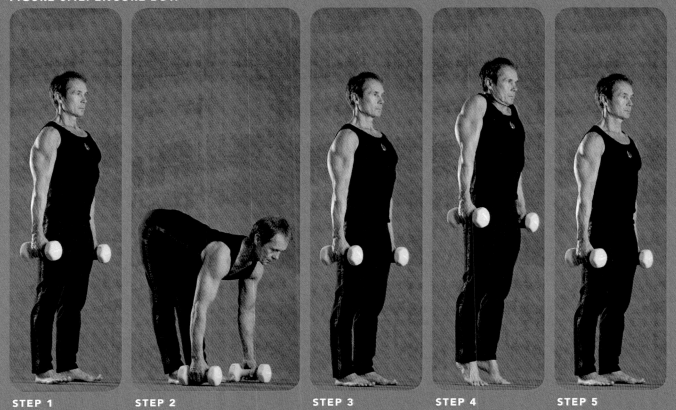

STEP 1   STEP 2   STEP 3   STEP 4   STEP 5

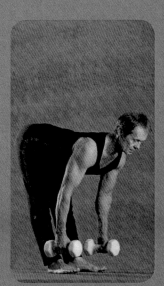

STEP 2a

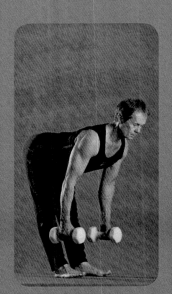

STEP 2b

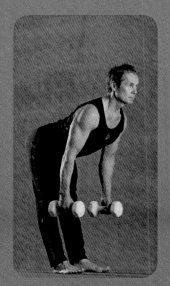

STEP 2c

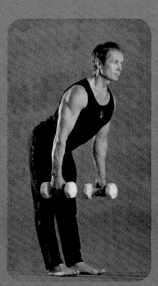

STEP 2d

SEQUENCE 1 ALL EXERCISES

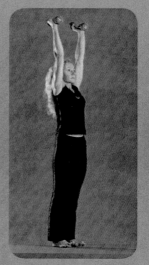

**SEQUENCE 1
EXERCISE 1**

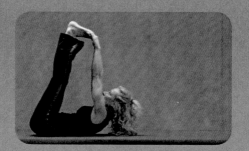

**SEQUENCE 1
EXERCISE 2**

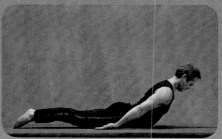

**SEQUENCE 1
EXERCISE 3**

SEQUENCE 2 ALL EXERCISES

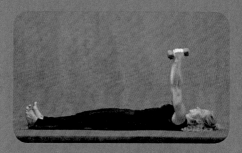

**SEQUENCE 2
EXERCISE 1**

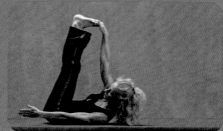

**SEQUENCE 2
EXERCISE 2**

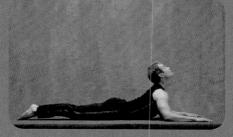

**SEQUENCE 2
EXERCISE 3**

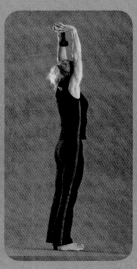

**SEQUENCE 1
EXERCISE 4**

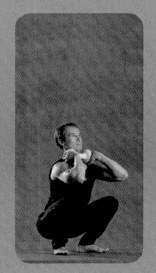

**SEQUENCE 1
EXERCISE 5**

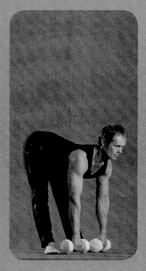

**SEQUENCE 1
EXERCISE 6**

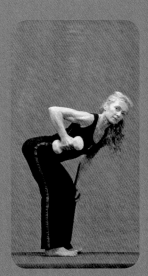

**SEQUENCE 2
EXERCISE 4**

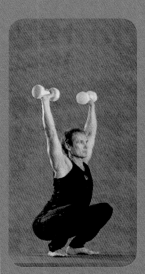

**SEQUENCE 2
EXERCISE 5**

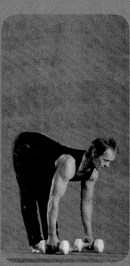

**SEQUENCE 2
EXERCISE 6**

It Cuts Through the BS to Simplicity and Ease

Jon Curry (44-year-old general contractor)

Boy, was I wrong about what makes and keeps you lean. I was a die-hard cyclist that believed I needed to be on the bike for hours, until it hurt, for it to be effective. As soon as I began The Happy Body program I immediately noticed an increase in energy, a better night's sleep, and an overall better attitude throughout the day. Jerzy and Aniela taught me how to stay healthy, save time, and feel the benefits of a muscle building workout and effective eating habits.

What I love most about The Happy Body program is the simplicity and ease. The workouts build core strength and flexibility without pushing your body for hours on end.

Aniela and Jerzy helped me to work through the everyday distractions of life and taught me how to make myself a priority. This has had an impact on every aspect of my life. I've gained back hours each day with this very livable, effective, and stress-free way to stay in shape and control my weight.

I am so thankful that I found Aniela and Jerzy and only wish everyone could have the fitness benefits of the program. It really works and cuts through the BS of all the time too often wasted on "trying" to be fit.

WEEK 3

REVIEWING YOUR FOOD PROGRAM

By the end of the second week, depending on your body type, you should have lost or gained 2% of your Ideal Body Weight.

If, however, in the second week alone, you lost more than 1% of your Ideal Body Weight, there is probably still some residual inflammation and bloating that are being worked off. On the other hand, if you are following the program precisely, you should not have lost less than 1% of your Ideal Body Weight during the second week.

If, in the second week alone, you gained more than 1% of your Ideal Body Weight, your muscles are still probably starved for nutrients and are absorbing water. On the other hand, if you are following the program precisely, you should not have gained less than 1% of your Ideal Body Weight during the second week.

REVIEWING YOUR EXERCISE PROGRAM

If, after performing Sequences 1 and 2 of the exercises for a week, your body or any part of it is sore or stiff, repeat the Sequences for the following week, but go down one level of difficulty in whatever exercises seem to be causing the problem. If you go all the way down to Level 1 and the problem persists, reduce the weight of your dumbbells by one pound until the problem ceases.

If your body or any part of it is not sore or stiff, and if the dumbbells you are lifting feel light, learn Sequence 3 of the exercises and perform them every day after you complete Sequences 1 and 2. In this case, however, instead of repeating the sequences four times, repeat each one three times.

For Exercises 3.1 through 3.6, follow the percentages given in Table 8.3.

For example, if you determined that you were comfortable lifting 2 pounds for Exercise 1.1, then, following Table 8.3, you will lift 3 pounds for Exercise 3.1, 1 pound for Exercise 3.4, 2 pounds for Exercise 3.5, and 3 pounds for Exercise 3.6.

PERFORM 3 SETS OF 6 REPETITIONS OF EVERY EXERCISE

TABLE 8.3: PERCENTAGES OF WEIGHT LIFTED IN SEQUENCES 1, 2, AND 3

SEQUENCE	EXERCISES					
	1	2	3	4	5	6
1	100%	na	na	150%	200%	150%
2	50%	na	na	200%	100%	150%
3	150%	na	na	50%	100%	150%

Lying Long

Description

Into the Exercise (positive lift)

Step 1: Place a dumbbell on the floor. Lie down face up with the dumbbell above your head, and take one end in each hand. Inhale deeply, then tighten your abdominal and buttocks muscles as you rotate your ankles and curl your toes toward your face.

Step 2: While holding your breath, lock your elbows and lift your arms straight up directly above your chest.

Step 3: Pause, stretch your arms further toward the ceiling, and hold.

Out of the Exercise (negative lift):

Step 4: In one continuous movement, release the stretch, return the dumbbell to the floor above your head, exhale as you unrotate your ankles and uncurl your toes, and release the tension in your abdominal and buttocks muscles.

Timing & Repetition

The total movement should take at least 10 seconds: 2 seconds for the inhale; 1 second for lifting the dumbbell; 1 second for the pause; 1 second for the stretch; 1 second for the hold; 2 seconds for lowering the dumbbell; and 2 seconds for the exhale and release. Repeat the exercise 6 times, which should take at least 60 seconds.

Purpose

This exercise has two purposes. First, it will strengthen your pectoral and lattissumus dorsi muscles ("lats"). Second, it will enhance the flexibility of your pectoral, rib cage, and shoulder muscles.

Levels of Difficulty

Level 1: Perform step 1d (elbows bent so that the dumbbell touches the top of the head), and then steps 2–4.

Level 2: Perform step 1c (elbows bent), and then steps 2–4.

Level 3: Perform step 1b (elbows slightly bent), and then steps 2–4.

Level 4: Perform step 1a (elbows unlocked), and then steps 2–4.

Level 5: Perform steps 1–4.

FIGURE 8.13: LYING LONG

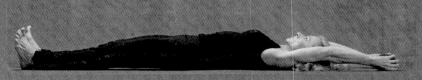

STEP 1

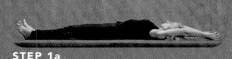

STEP 1a

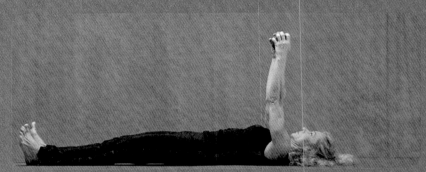

STEP 2

STEP 1b

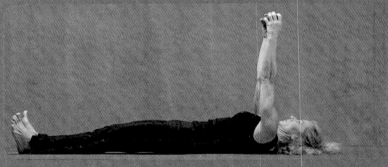

STEP 3

STEP 1c

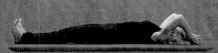

STEP 1d

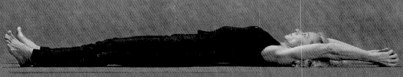

STEP 4

Rolling Wave

Description

Into the Exercise (positive lift)

Step 1: Lie flat on your back with your arms stretched out above your head. Inhale deeply, then tighten your abdominal muscles as you rotate your ankles and curl your toes toward your face.

Steps 2 & 3: In one continuous movement, raise your arms and head off the floor, rounding your back as you lift up one vertebra at a time until you touch your toes while arching your back.

Step 4: Stretch your arms another inch or two past your toes while arching your back slightly more.

Out of the Exercise (negative lift)

Step 5: In one continuous movement, release the stretch and round your back, then return to your original position, lowering your back one vertebra at a time. As you exhale, unrotate your ankles, uncurl your toes, and release the tension in your abdominal muscles.

Timing & Repetition

The total movement should take at least 10 seconds: 2 seconds for the inhale; 2 seconds for the positive lift; 1 second for the pause; 1 second for the stretch; 1 second for the hold; 1 second for the negative lift; and 2 seconds for the exhale. Repeat the exercise 6 times, which should take at least 60 seconds.

Purpose

This exercise has two purposes. First, it will strengthen your abdominal muscles. Second, it will enhance the flexibility of your hips and back.

Levels of Difficulty

Level 1: Perform steps 1 and 3c (raise your shoulders off the floor and point your fingers toward the ceiling). Then perform step 5.

Level 2: Perform steps 1, 2, and 3b (touch your knees instead of your toes as you arch your back). Then perform step 5.

Level 3: Perform steps 1, 2, and 3a (touch your shins instead of your toes as you arch your back). Then perform step 5.

Level 4: Perform steps 1, 2, 3, and 5.

Level 5: Perform steps 1–5.

FIGURE 8.14: ROLLING WAVE

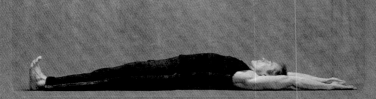

STEP 1

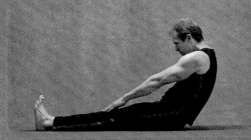

STEP 2

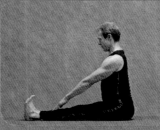

STEP 3a

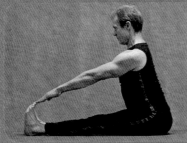

STEP 3

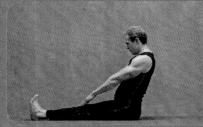

STEP 3b

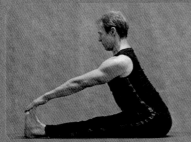

STEP 4

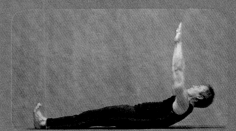

STEP 3c

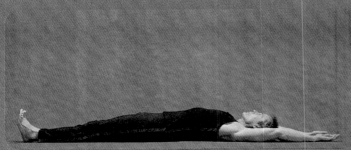

STEP 5

3   3   Lift Off

Description

Into the Exercise (positive lift)

Step 1: Lie on your belly with your arms at your side, your palms facing up, and your head facing to the one side. Inhale deeply, then tighten your abdominal, buttocks, and hamstring muscles.

Step 2: Keeping your arms relaxed and your hands and feet touching the floor, raise your upper body and lift your face upward until you see the ceiling. Pause for one second.

Step 3: Raise your upper body another inch or two by lifting slightly more off the floor at the waist.

Out of the Exercise (negative lift)

Step 4: In one continuous movement, lower your upper body to the floor, turning your head toward the opposite direction, and then exhale as you relax your abdominal, buttocks, and hamstring muscles.

Timing & Repetition

The total movement should take at least 8 seconds: 2 seconds for the inhale; 1 second for raising the body; 1 second for the pause; 1 second for the extension; 1 second for lowering the body; and 2 seconds for the exhale and release. Repeat the exercise 6 times, which should take at least 48 seconds.

Purpose

This exercise has three purposes. First, it will strengthen your lumbar, thoracic, and cervical muscles. Second, it will enhance the flexibility of your neck and rib cage. Third, it will enhance your neck's range of motion by stretching your trapezius, sternocleidomastoid, and related muscles.

Levels of Difficulty

Level 1: Perform steps 1 and 2c (keeping your arms relaxed and your hands and feet touching the floor, raise your upper body and head off the floor just enough to look down at the floor). Then perform step 4.

Level 2: Perform steps 1 and 2b (keeping your arms relaxed and your hands and feet touching the floor, raise your upper body and head off the floor several feet ahead of you). Then perform step 4.

Level 3: Perform steps 1 and 2a (keeping your arms relaxed and your hands and feet touching the floor, raise your upper body and head off the floor several feet ahead of you). Then perform step 4.

Level 4: Perform steps 1, 2, and 4.

Level 5: Perform steps 1–4.

FIGURE 8.15: LIFT OFF

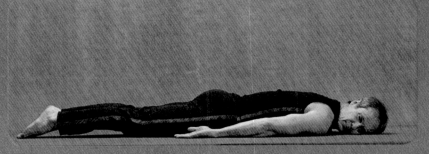

STEP 1

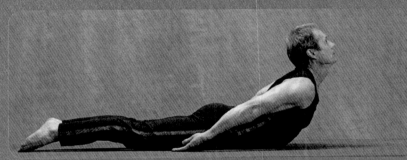

STEP 2

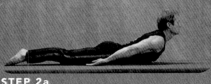

STEP 2a

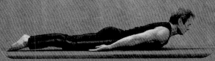

STEP 2b

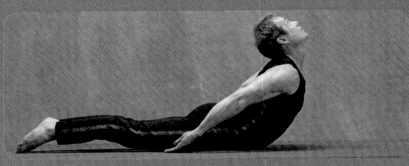

STEP 3

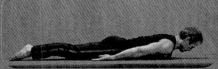

STEP 2c

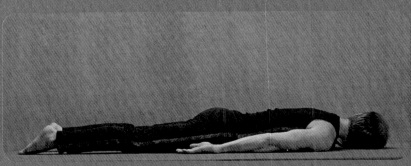

STEP 4

Working Hinges

Description

Into the Exercise (positive lift)

Step 1: Take a dumbbell in each hand, and stand upright with your feet directly under your hips with arms hanging straight down at your sides. Lift your chest and take a deep breath, then curl up your toes and tighten your abdominal and buttocks muscles.

Steps 2, 3, & 4: While holding your breath, lift your hands 90 degrees in front of you so that your arms are parallel to the ground, without moving your elbows backward. Rotate your wrists so that your palms face up. Then, keeping your elbows pressed against your ribs, move your hands outward 90 degrees to the 3:00 o'clock position.

Step 5: Pause and shift your weight totally back onto your heels, simultaneously moving your hands slightly backward. Hold your balance for one second.

Out of the Exercise (negative lift):

Steps 6, 7, & 8: In one continuous movement, release the stretch and return your feet to their normal position with your toes still curled; bring your hands inward 90 degrees without moving your elbows backward, then rotate your wrists so that your palms face each other. Lower the dumbbells to your sides and exhale as you uncurl your toes and release the tension in your abdominal and buttocks muscles.

Timing & Repetition

The total movement should take at least 11 seconds: 2 seconds for the inhale; 2 seconds for lifting the dumbbells; 1 second for the pause; 1 second for the stretch; 1 second for the hold; 2 seconds for lowering the dumbbells; and 2 seconds for the exhale and release. Repeat the exercise 6 times, which should take at least 66 seconds.

Purpose

This exercise has three purposes. First, it will strengthen your rear deltoid muscles by your lifting heavier weights over time. Second, it will improve the flexibility of your rotary cuffs. Third, it will improve your balance by shifting your weight totally onto your heels.

Levels of Difficulty

Level 1: Perform steps 1–3 and 4c (moving your hands outward only slightly). Then perform steps 6–8.

Level 2: Perform steps 1–3 and 4b (moving your hands outward only to the 1:00 o'clock position). Then perform steps 6–8.

Level 3: Perform steps 1–3 and 4a (moving your hands outward only to the 2:00 o'clock position). Then perform steps 6–8.

Level 4: Perform steps 1–4, 6–8.

Level 5: Perform steps 1–8.

FIGURE 8.16: WORKING HINGES

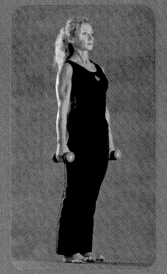

STEP 1

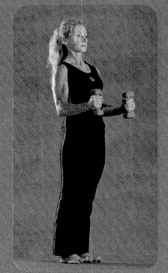

STEP 2

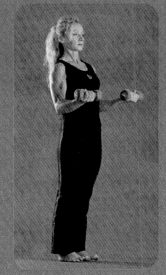

STEP 3

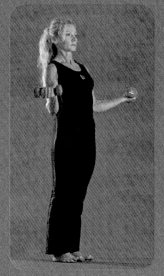

STEP 4

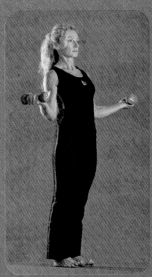

STEP 5

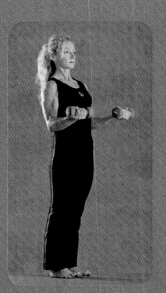

STEP 6

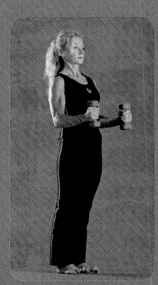

STEP 7

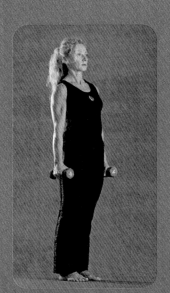

STEP 8

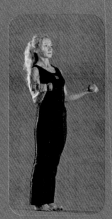

STEP 4a

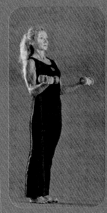

STEP 4b

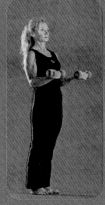

STEP 4c

SEQUENCE 3 · EXERCISE 5 · Power Tower

Description

Into the Exercise (positive lift)

Step 1: Holding dumbbells at your sides, stand with your feet a shoulder length apart and your toes pointed outward. Lift your chest and inhale deeply, then flex your abdominal muscles and curl your toes upward.

Steps 2, 3, & 4: In a continuous motion, without moving your elbows backward, lift the dumbbells parallel to each other until they are at chin level, then rotate your arms backward.

Steps 5, 6, & 7: Squat without bending forward or raising your heels. While in the squat position, press the dumbbells above your head until your elbows lock. Then immediately stand up straight.

Out of the Exercise (negative lift):

Steps 8, 9, 10, & 11: In a continuous movement, lower the dumbbells to chin level; rotate your arms forward; and lower your arms to the starting position without moving your elbows backward. Then exhale as you relax your abdominal muscles and uncurl your toes.

Timing & Repetition

The total movement should take at least 9 seconds: 2 seconds for the inhale; 1 second for the squat; 1 second for the press; 1 second for standing up; 2 seconds for lowering the dumbbells; and 2 seconds for the exhale and release. Repeat the exercise 6 times, which should take at least 54 seconds.

Purpose

This exercise has three purposes. First, it will strengthen your thigh, buttock, lower back, and deltoid muscles. Second, it will improve the flexibility of your ankles, knees, hips, spine, shoulders, and wrists. Third, it will enhance your posture and balance by forcing your spine to arch backward throughout the exercise.

Levels of Difficulty

Level 1: Perform steps 1–4, 5d (squatting slightly), and 6–11.

Level 2: Using a low table or bench, perform steps 1–4, 5c, and 6–11.

Level 3: Using a low table or bench, perform steps 1–4, 5b, and 6–11.

Level 4: Using a low table or bench, perform steps 1–4, 5a, and 6–11.

Level 5: Perform steps 1–11.

SEQUENCE 3, EXERCISE 5

FIGURE 8.17: POWER TOWER

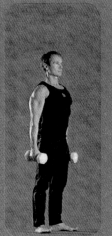 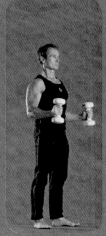 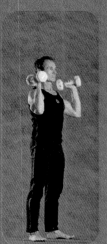 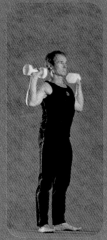 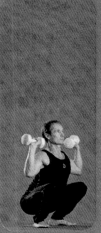 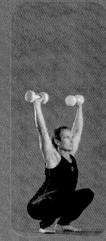

STEP 1 STEP 2 STEP 3 STEP 4 STEP 5 STEP 6

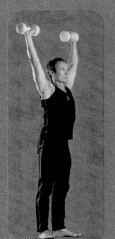 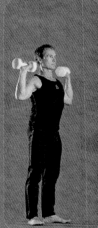 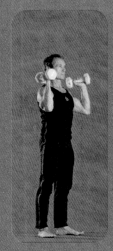 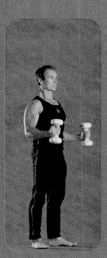 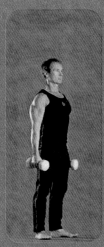

STEP 7 STEP 8 STEP 9 STEP 10 STEP 11

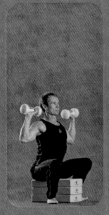 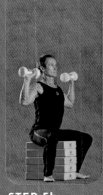 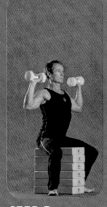 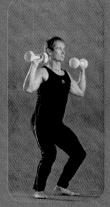

STEP 5a STEP 5b STEP 5c STEP 5d

SEQUENCE 3 | EXERCISE 6 | Final Bow

Description

Into the Exercise (positive lift)

Step 1: Take a dumbbell in each hand, and stand upright with your feet together with arms hanging straight down at your sides. Lift your chest and take a deep breath, then curl up your toes, lock your knees, and tighten your abdominal muscles.

Step 2: While holding your breath and keeping your knees locked, bend forward till the dumbbells touch the ground.

Step 3: Without pausing, stand up straight and tighten your buttocks muscles.

Step 4: Stand on your toes and simultaneously rotate your shoulders backward and upward, holding this pose for two seconds.

Out of the Exercise (negative lift):

Step 5: In one continuous movement, release the stretch, return your feet to the starting position, and exhale as you release the tension in your abdominal and buttocks muscles.

Timing & Repetition

The total movement should take at least 10 seconds: 2 seconds for the inhale; 1 second for bending forward; 1 second for the lift; 1 second for the stretch; 2 seconds for the hold; 1 second for lowering your shoulders and heels, and 2 seconds for the exhale and release. Repeat the exercise 6 times, which should take at least 60 seconds.

Purpose

This exercise has three purposes. First, it will strengthen your hamstrings and lower back. Second, it will improve the flexibility of your trapezium muscles, spine, hamstrings, and calves. Third, it will improve your balance by shifting your weight totally onto your toes.

Levels of Difficulty

Level 1: Perform steps 1, 2d (mid-thigh level), 3, 4, and 5.

Level 2: Perform steps 1, 2c (knee level), 3, 4, and 5.

Level 3: Perform steps 1, 2b (mid-shin level), 3, 4, and 5.

Level 4: Perform steps 1, 2a (ankle level), 3, 4, and 5.

Level 5: Perform steps 1–5.

FIGURE 8.18: FINAL BOW

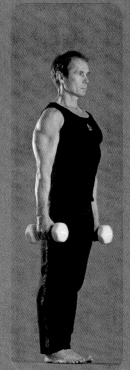

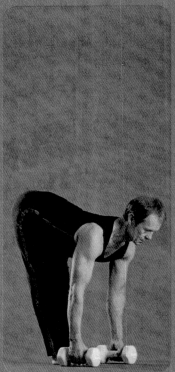

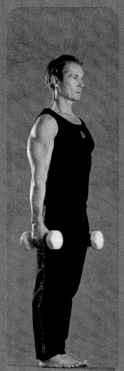

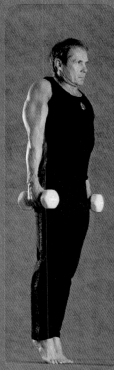

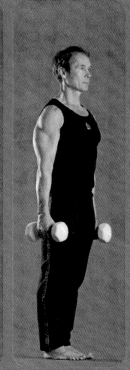

STEP 1   STEP 2   STEP 3   STEP 4   STEP 5

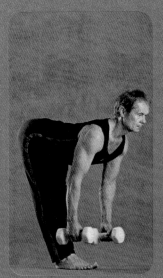

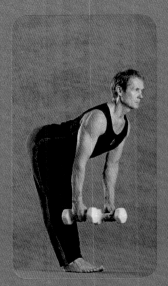

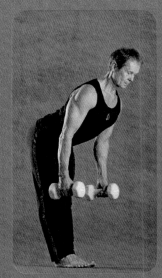

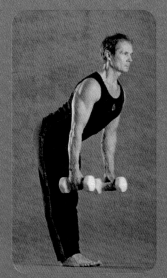

STEP 2a   STEP 2b   STEP 2c   STEP 2d

SEQUENCE 1 ALL EXERCISES

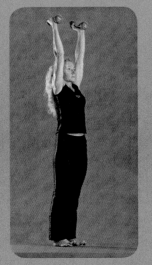

**SEQUENCE 1
EXERCISE 1**

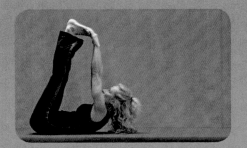

**SEQUENCE 1
EXERCISE 2**

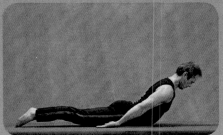

**SEQUENCE 1
EXERCISE 3**

SEQUENCE 2 ALL EXERCISES

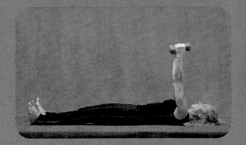

**SEQUENCE 2
EXERCISE 1**

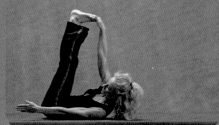

**SEQUENCE 2
EXERCISE 2**

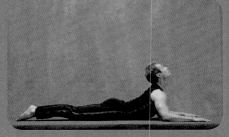

**SEQUENCE 2
EXERCISE 3**

SEQUENCE 3 ALL EXERCISES

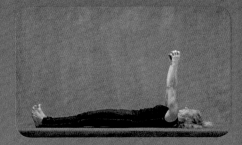

**SEQUENCE 3
EXERCISE 1**

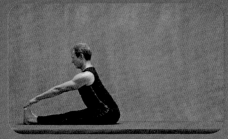

**SEQUENCE 3
EXERCISE 2**

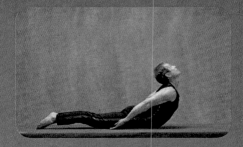

**SEQUENCE 3
EXERCISE 3**

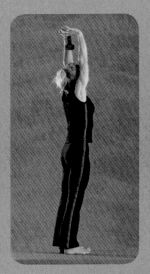

**SEQUENCE 1
EXERCISE 4**

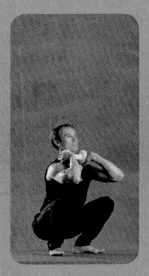

**SEQUENCE 1
EXERCISE 5**

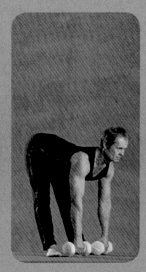

**SEQUENCE 1
EXERCISE 6**

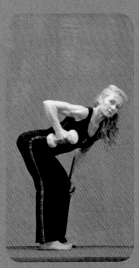

**SEQUENCE 2
EXERCISE 4**

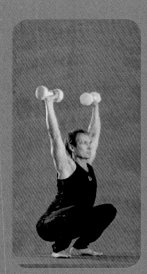

**SEQUENCE 2
EXERCISE 5**

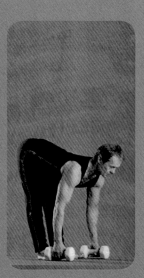

**SEQUENCE 2
EXERCISE 6**

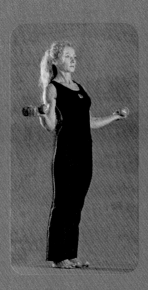

**SEQUENCE 3
EXERCISE 4**

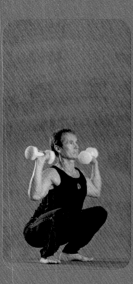

**SEQUENCE 3
EXERCISE 5**

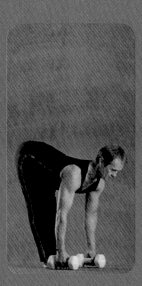

**SEQUENCE 3
EXERCISE 6**

The Long Ball

Andrew Buchanan (13-year-old student)

I started doing the Happy Body program after my mom and sister had been doing it for the first two months of summer. My mom told me that it would help me gain muscle and do better in golf and baseball. At the time, I was on a traveling baseball team and played in golf competitions all over the state.

The first time I met them, we talked about my eating habits and how they could change. I felt that I ate well, however they told me that I should not have any bread as they are unproductive carbohydrates. Also, I ate a lot for breakfast, lunch, and dinner, and I exercised, but I never gained any muscle. They told me that I needed to have six meals including three meals of a power bar or another type of snack. Also, I started a 45-minute work-out program consisting of lifting weights, squatting, and jumping. At the end of the workout, I meditate for five minutes, which gives me a chance to relax and take everything off my mind.

Since I started, I have lost 5 pounds of fat and gained 15 pounds of muscle, and I am now 107 pounds. Before, when playing golf, I was able to hit the ball somewhat far. I usually hit 220 yards on average, and my longest drives were around 250 yards. After just four months of working with Aniela and Jerzy, I started to hit the ball on average 250 yards, and I hit a long ball of 300 yards.

Jerzy and Aniela have helped me become healthier and happier. I have improved in golf and become stronger. The workout is something that I will continue to do for the rest of my life.

CHAPTER 8: LEARNING THE EXERCISES

WEEK 4

Reviewing Your Food Program

By the end of the third week, depending on your body type, you should have lost or gained 3% of your Ideal Body Weight.

If, however, in the third week alone, you lost more than 1% of your Ideal Body Weight, you must be undereating, and therefore you are in danger of burning muscle instead of fat. If so, the warning signs will include lightheadedness, slugglishness, fatigue, and muscle soreness. The most obvious warning sign, however, will be hunger pangs. In that case, you will likely begin to overeat in compensation, and that will jeopardize your achieving your desired body. To correct this, increase every snack by 10 calories for the next week and see if you have stopped losing more than 1% of your Ideal Body Weight for that week. If not, repeat this increase weekly until you have achieved the proper loss.

If, in the third week alone, you gained more than 1% of your Ideal Body Weight, you must be overeating. In that case, you need to decrease every snack by 10 calories for the next week and see if you have stopped gaining more than 1% of your Ideal Body Weight for that week. If not, repeat this decrease weekly until you have achieved the proper loss.

Reviewing Your Exercise Program

If, after performing Sequences 1, 2, and 3 of the exercises for a week, your body or any part of it is sore or stiff, repeat the Sequences for the following week, but go down one level of difficulty in whatever exercises seem to be causing the problem. If you go all the way down to Level 1 and the problem persists, reduce the weight of your dumbbells by one pound until the problem ceases.

If your body or any part of it is not sore or stiff, and if the dumbbells you are lifting feel comfortable, you are ready to begin increasing the weight of the dumbbells by recalculating the weight for Exercise 1.1 and then following the percentages in Table 8.3 (page 149).

WEEKS 5 AND 6

Reviewing Your Food Program

By the end of the fourth week, depending on your body type, you should have lost or gained 4% of your Ideal Body Weight. By the end of the fifth week, depending on your body type, you should have lost or gained 5% of your Ideal Body Weight, and your eating habits should be stable.

Reviewing Your Exercise Program

If your body or any part of it is not sore or stiff, and if the dumbbells you are lifting feel comfortable, you can again increase the weight of the dumbbells by recalculating the weight for Exercise 1.1 and then following the percentages in Table 8.3. By now, you should be sleeping better, waking up refreshed, having more energy during the day, feeling more relaxed, and experiencing less or no physical pain.

WEEK 7

Reviewing Your Food Program

By the end of the sixth week, depending on your body type, you should have lost or gained 6% of your Ideal Body Weight, and you should be feeling more youthful. If you have met these goals, continue your food plan unchanged until you have achieved your Ideal Body Weight and Ideal Body Weight Proportions. At that point, you begin your maintenance program. In order to stop losing any more weight, you must eat more than you have been eating up to now. To calculate how much more, you need to calculate how many calories equal 1% of your Ideal Body Weight and add that number of calories to your daily intake of food.

For example, if an overweight woman's Ideal Body Weight is 110 pounds, she was losing 1.1 pounds of fat every week, which is equal to 3,850 calories per week, or 550 calories per day. Thus, she should now add 550 calories to her daily intake.

    1 pound of fat = 3,500 calories
    1.1 pound of fat = 3,850 calories ÷ 7 = 550

The best way to do this is to eat bigger portions of vegetables and proteins for your meals and increase the size of your snacks. If you like to have an alcoholic beverage with your meals, be sure to do it with vegetables. If you are craving some foods that you have eliminated from your diet, consider bringing them back in measured doses, one by one, and see the result at the end of every week.

If an underweight woman of the same height had been gaining weight at a rate of 1.1 pounds every week, she should deduct 550 calories from her daily intake after she achieves her Ideal Body Weight.

It is acceptable to oscillate 2% above or below your Ideal Body Weight. Thus, the women in the above examples may maintain their Ideal Body Weights by staying between 108 and 112 pounds. If their weight drops below 108 pounds, they should increase their food intake, and if their weight rises above 112 pounds, they should decrease their food intake.

Reviewing Your Exercise Program

By the end of the sixth week, the exercises should have become so familiar to you that you can complete them in 40 to 50 minutes. Once you have mastered every movement, you should be able to accelerate the workout until eventually it is so second nature that you can complete the whole cycle in 30 minutes. When that is the case, men should increase the weight they lift by 2 pounds, and women should increase it by 1 pound. Do this until your body adapts to the new weights and you are comfortable with all 18 exercises. Keep increasing the weights in this way until you have achieved all six of The Happy Body Standards. From that point on, you will have a youthful body and will only need to maintain it.

By the end of the sixth week, depending on your body type, you should have lost or gained 6% of your Ideal Body Weight, and you should be feeling more youthful.

A Habit, Like Brushing Your Teeth Everyday

Faye Mellos (52-year-old financial advisor)

One spring I noticed my friend Betty just kept looking better and better every time I saw her. Finally she told me what she was doing in hopes that I could get my extremely overweight husband into shape. She had been working with Jerzy and Aniela's Happy Body program. I thought about it and figured if I went first, my husband might then be willing to go, too.

When I first arrived at Jerzy and Aniela's home the first thought that went through my mind was, "This isn't a gym. What's up with this?" First rule when I arrived: Kick off your shoes.

I sat down in the den with Jerzy, Aniela, and a hot cup of tea and started a fantastic journey toward having a happy body. At first the whole idea of The Happy Body sounded so trite, but I have to say after about 30 days of light weight lifting and eating right, my body started talking back to me. If I ate food that was not "good fuel" for me, my body let me know. If I ate the right food, I really felt like my body was "happy."

The weight lifting and stretching is a whole other issue. At first I thought, "How stupid is this to do 30 minutes of light weights and stretches? Dumb, dumb, dumb." But I kept reminding myself that Betty looked great, and every time I saw her she seemed a little younger. So, I thought, for the money and time I should just suck it up, and do it. If it didn't work I could quit at anytime.

A year before meeting Jerzy and Aniela I had purchased a road bike and spent 3 days each week in an endurance cycling class, riding two hours per session. I thought I was in pretty good shape, except that during that year of regular endurance cycling I gained 8 pounds and damaged one of my knees to the point where I could hardly walk. I knew that this was not working, but what else could I do?

It is funny when I think about it all. The endurance cycling center had a lot of sophisticated machines to hook you up to after each 3-month session and give you your percentage of body fat and level of endurance. It was all very impressive, and I never questioned what the trainers said or told me to do.

The first day of The Happy Body program Jerzy pulled out a bikini and said: "Put it on; time for pictures." I was horrified but went along. He measured a few places on my body, took my pictures, and ended up with the exact same results as the high-tech gadgets at the cycling club.

After a week of light lifting for only 30 minutes each day, listening to music afterwards for 5 minutes, and giving up the guilt of not going to the gym, I dropped both my gym and my endurance cycling memberships. I did not feel guilty doing it, as I knew then that I didn't need those memberships to be strong and healthy. Basically, all I needed were a few free weights, some space on the floor, and I was in business.

I went from a tight-fitting size 12 to a perfect size 6 in just 9 months and I'm currently holding steady. I have been at this weight many times before but never at this size. I am toned and feel very strong. My body and level of fitness have changed from what I thought was not so bad to very good. I still have a ways to go, but I don't feel the frenzy of having to do it all today. One of the first things that stuck with me was when Jerzy told me, "This will become a habit, like brushing your teeth." He was right. Now if I don't lift everyday, something feels out of synch. I feel just like I would if I didn't brush my teeth. I am not perfect yet, but I trust myself that I will eventually get there and reach my goal. I have all the tools I need right in my own home.

Charting Your Progress

Every six weeks, you should record your body measurement progress. For example, if you are a 5'2" woman who initially weighs 146 pounds, of which 42% (61.32 lbs) is fat, you need to gain 11.02 pounds of muscle and lose 47.02 pounds of fat, which will take you 50.09 weeks (see the calculations for this in Body Type 7, page 90).

TABLE 8.4: SAMPLE OF BODY WEIGHT PROPORTION MEASUREMENTS FOR A 5'2" WOMAN

	Date	Body Fat (%)	Body Weight (pounds)	Muscle Weight (pounds)	Fat Weight (pounds)
Baseline	4-11-07	42%	146.2	84.8	61.4
Week 6		38%	137.7	85.4	52.3
Week 12		34%	131.8	87.7	44.1
Week 18		29%	124.1	88.2	35.9
Week 24		24%	117.8	89.5	28.3
Week 30		19%	112.2	90.9	21.3
Week 36		17%	110.9	92.1	18.8
Week 42		15%	111.1	94.4	16.7
Week 48		14%	110.3	94.9	15.4
Week 54		13%	109.7	95.4	14.3
Ideal		**13%**			

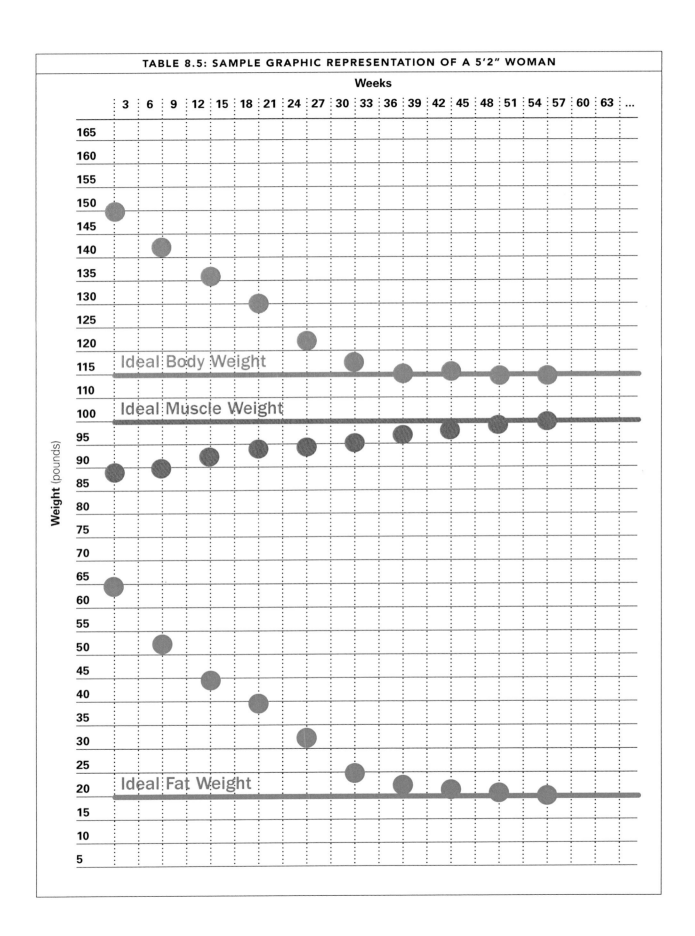

TABLE 8.5: SAMPLE GRAPHIC REPRESENTATION OF A 5'2" WOMAN

Using Table 8.6 and Table 8.7, chart your own progress.

	Date	Body Fat (%)	Body Weight (pounds)	Muscle Weight (pounds)	Fat Weight (pounds)
TABLE 8.6: PROGRESS OF YOUR BODY WEIGHT PROPORTION MEASUREMENTS					
Baseline					
Week 6					
Week 12					
Week 18					
Week 24					
Week 30					
Week 36					
Week 42					
Week 48					
Week 54					
Ideal					

TABLE 8.7: GRAPHIC REPRESENTATION OF YOUR PROGRESS

Weeks

Weight (pounds)	3	6	9	12	15	18	21	24	27	30	33	36	39	42	45	48	51	54	57	60	63	...
300																						
290																						
280																						
270																						
260																						
250																						
240																						
230																						
220																						
210																						
200																						
190																						
180																						
170																						
160																						
150																						
140																						
130																						
120																						
110																						
100																						
90																						
80																						
70																						
60																						
50																						
40																						
30																						
20																						
10																						
0																						

COPY THIS FORM FOR YOUR OWN PERSONAL USE

Reviewing The Happy Body Standards

Every six weeks, you should grade your youthfulness on a scale of 1 to 5:

1 = poor
2 = fair
3 = good
4 = very good
5 = excellent

Before you test yourself for the Standard of Speed, you must have achieved a score of excellent in the Standard of Strength.

Example 1 (before achieving 5 on Standard of Strength). Refer to Table 8.8:

1 + 2 + 2 + 3 + 1 + 1 + 1 + 1 + 3 = 15
Then, 15 ÷ 9 = 1.7

Example 2 (after achieving 5 on Standard of Strength). Refer to Table 8.9:

3 + 4 + 4 + 5 + 4 + 5 + 1 + 4 + 5 + 5 = 40
Then, 40 ÷ 10 = 4.0

TABLE 8.8: SAMPLE OF TESTING YOUTHFULNESS

| | Table | Flexibility | | | | Strength | Speed | Leanness | Ideal Body Weight | Good Posture | Grade |
		Jack Knife	Bow	Cork Screw	Candle Squat						
Week 6	1	2	2	3	1	1	—	1	1	3	1.7

TABLE 8.9: SAMPLE OF TESTING YOUTHFULNESS

| | Table | Flexibility | | | | Strength | Speed | Leanness | Ideal Body Weight | Good Posture | Grade |
		Jack Knife	Bow	Cork Screw	Candle Squat						
Week 42	3	4	4	5	4	5	1	4	5	5	4.0

Using Table 8.10, keep track of your own progress.

		Flexibility			Strength	Speed	Leanness	Ideal Body Weight	Good Posture	Grade
	Table	Jack Knife	Bow	Cork Screw	Candle Squat					
Week 6										
Week 12										
Week 18										
Week 24										
Week 30										
Week 36										
Week 42										
Week 48										
Week 54										
Week 60										
Week 66										
Week 72										
Week 78										
Week 84										
Week 90										
Week 96										
Week 102										
Week 108										
Week 114										
Week 120										

TABLE 8.10: TESTING YOUR YOUTHFULNESS

COPY THIS FORM FOR YOUR OWN PERSONAL USE

Reviewing Your Progress in Pictures

Every time you have lost 6% of your Ideal Body Weight (for most people, every six weeks), take three full-body photographs of yourself in a brief bathing suit (bikini for women)—front, back, and side—and one frontal close-up photograph of your face from the shoulders up.

Arrange the photographs as in Figure 8.19, below, to observe your progress in body shape and posture. Looking at the first week of pictures will encourage you to never want that body again and will motivate you to continue toward your goal. When you have achieved it, the pictures will inspire you to keep the best body you've ever had.

FIGURE 8.19: YOUR PROGRESS IN PICTURES

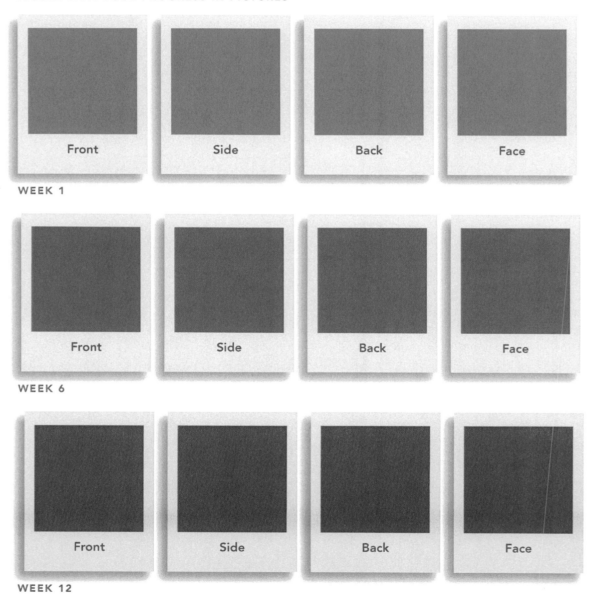

WEEK 1 — Front, Side, Back, Face

WEEK 6 — Front, Side, Back, Face

WEEK 12 — Front, Side, Back, Face

The Dreaded Mid-Life Crisis

Robyn Rajkovich (51-year-old administrator)

I came upon Jerzy and Aniela by fate. One day I was in the nail salon, hearing about these incredible trainers to the stars who transform lives. The next thing I knew, I was on the phone talking to Jerzy, the man behind The Happy Body program. I tried to hold off meeting with him because I had a hunch he wouldn't be happy with my current physical state. I politely said, "Thank you. I will think about it and call you." I was surprised when he replied, "No, you will come see me tomorrow at 3:00 pm."

I had recently seen the break-up of my 24-year marriage and suffered from a bout with ovarian cancer, resulting in a hysterectomy. I had been diagnosed with painful fibromyalgia years earlier and dealt with that through medication. I had difficulty sleeping, which exacerbated my symptoms. I had long been the endless giver — one who took care of everyone around me but never made time for myself. I had a high-stress job, two daughters, and everything seemed out-of-balance. I was in a rut. I was emotionally and physically exhausted. Tomorrow? Okay, I thought, what do I have to lose?

The next day, I showed up for the meeting and — I have to be honest here — was immediately intimidated. Jerzy is not a large man in physical terms, but he has a very large presence. However, it didn't take long to realize he's probably one of the warmest and kindest men I had ever met. He's also frank and to the point. I was definitely not prepared when he said, "Here, go with Aniela. She will give you one of her bathing suits to change into so I can get some pictures of you."

Needless to say, I just about fell to the floor. Here was Aniela, the female version of Jerzy. With her perfect body, how was I going to get into her bathing suit? And then, how was I supposed to come out and have my pictures taken by this stranger?

I got into the swimsuit, but honestly think I stayed in the bathroom for an extra twenty minutes trying to decide if I should open the door or climb out the window and drive away. I finally decided that driving away was probably futile because I was sure he would hunt me down, so I took a deep breath and opened the door.

Right then and there, I began to leave my old self behind.

Over the following weeks I was taught exercise, controlled eating, meditation, and stretching, and how to incorporate them into my chaotic daily life. As I did, everything seemed to change – some seemingly overnight. I felt better about myself,

[CONTINUED ON NEXT PAGE]

physically and emotionally. I made sure to make time for me and to gain control over those things that bring me stress.

The Happy Body program transformed my life in every conceivable way. Now, four years later, I find myself full of energy; I'm healthier and happier than I've ever been before. I ended up marrying the man of my dreams who brought to my life the bonus package of five amazing, beautiful children. Life couldn't have worked out more perfectly, and I can't thank Jerzy and Aniela enough for helping me turn my life around.

I wholeheartedly recommend The Happy Body program to others like me. It's time to change your priorities and make The Happy Body program part of your life, just as I did mine. It definitely made me a healthier person physically, emotionally, and spiritually in ways I never could have imagined.

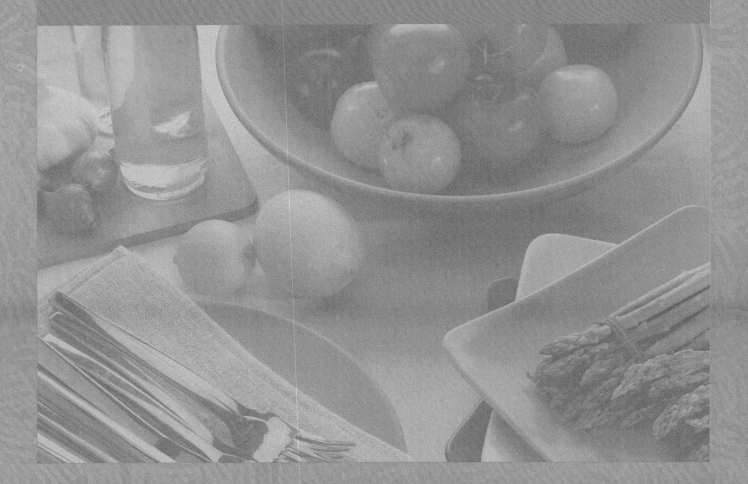

NOURISHING YOUR HAPPY BODY

PART 3

INTO
THE
KITCHEN

THE HAPPY BELLY

Competing in Olympic weightlifting requires us to eat nutritious food. Our goal is to perform at our absolute best, which means that we have to choose quality food that helps us to lower our percentage of body fat and maintain our muscle size, while improving our performance and recovery.

Over the years, we have tried many different diets in the search for optimal nutrition to support health as well as top athletic performance. As our experience below demonstrates, any diet, when taken to the extreme can be dangerous.

Until the early 1980s, we ate a balanced American diet. But then we started to meditate, and that led us to a spiritual path. Soon we were eating only raw vegetables, fruits, and nuts. Unfortunately, after a year on that diet, we started to have problems that we had never experienced before on a regular basis, such as migraine headaches, stomach cramps, diarrhea, constipation, bloating, and sluggishness. At first, we assumed that our bodies would adapt to the new diet, but they did not. Even worse, we saw that our weightlifting performance was declining. We could no longer match our personal best records.

Then Jerzy began to develop itchy eyes. Even prescription eye drops didn't help. The itching

got worse than ever, and Jerzy started to develop breathing problems.

An allergy specialist suggested that the problem might be mold or pollen, so we sealed all the windows, sterilized the inside of the house, and put air purifiers in all the rooms. All of that made no difference.

Next, a pulmonary specialist diagnosed Jerzy with asthma and prescribed an antihistamine medication. The symptoms went away, but Jerzy progressively felt weaker.

Blood tests revealed that Jerzy was anemic, so he starting taking iron supplements. However, he developed severe abdominal pains for which he underwent numerous tests, including a colonoscopy, an upper gastrointestinal barium test, and a CT scan. They were negative, and the pains persisted.

Then a friend suggested a holistic doctor, who analyzed Jerzy's saliva and determined that he had fungi throughout his digestive system. He prescribed a solution of liquid silver to kill the fungi and also advised Jerzy to resume cooking his food. Like everything else, this did no good whatsoever.

On top of everything else, Jerzy noticed that his fingernails and toenails were unusually soft. At that point, his regular chiropractor suggested that the problems might be caused by Jerzy's raw diet and advised him to go back to eating red meat. Even so, the chiropractor warned it could take a year or two for him to recover.

However, Jerzy did not immediately return to red meat because he thought he had a protein deficiency. So, looking for vegetarian sources of protein, he began eating tofu, beans, and rice. After three months, feeling no difference, he gave up on pure vegetarianism by adding egg whites and milk products—including cheese, cottage cheese, and yogurt—back to his diet. Still seeing no progress, he returned to eating animal protein—first fish and then chicken.

It took a year for Jerzy to get off antihistamine medication. He would stop it for a while and then take it again when the itching and the asthma returned. Eventually, after two years, just as the chiropractor had predicted, the itching and the breathing problems totally disappeared. A blood test confirmed that Jerzy was also no longer anemic. The soft nails hardened, but became coarse and brittle—the only effect of a taken-to-the-extreme raw diet that has remained to this day.

Throughout this period, by the way, Aniela had none of these problems, aside from her declining weightlifting performance. Nevertheless, after watching what had happened to Jerzy and listening to vegetarian clients who were having similar problems, she decided to also resume eating red meat.

Many years later, while working with vegans and vegetarians who had weight problems, Jerzy came to realize that his problem was not his vegetarianism

but his consumption of man-made food products. Within Jerzy's limitations of not wanting to gain weight while also supporting top athletic performance, processed foods simply didn't provide enough nutrition. This compromised his immune system, which led to his health problems.

Today authors warn us that gluten, saturated fat, or protein can cause the same diseases: osteoporosis, heart attack, stroke, cancer, diabetes, brain disorders, and more. If we eliminate one ingredient from our diet, then we eat too much of the other and expose ourselves to more danger. It seems that the only way out is eating complete meals. Thus, whether or not one is a vegetarian, it is essential to eat sufficient amounts of protein, vegetables, fruit, and nuts in their natural state.

On our diet discovery journey, Table 9.1 includes the foods we have found that are the best high-protein sources.

TABLE 9.1: SOURCES OF HIGH PROTEIN	
Animal Proteins	**Plant Proteins**
Beef	Spinach
Buffalo	Tofu
Lamb	Soy Beans
Veal	Broccoli
Ostrich	Oat Bran
Pork	Peas (all)
Chicken Legs	Beans (all)
Turkey Legs	Whole Wheat
Chicken Breast	Peanuts
Turkey Breast	Quinoa
Fish	Almonds
Egg Whites	Bulgur
Cheese (low-fat)	Couscous

COMPLETE MEALS

We want people to always eat complete meals. By complete, we mean a mixture of protein and vegetables in the proper proportions. These meals can come in several different forms, including:

- soups & stews
- salads
- omelets, soufflés & other egg white dishes
- free-choice dinners (protein dishes and vegetable dishes)

Each of the first three categories above constitutes a complete meal, containing protein and vegetables. Therefore, you cannot have more than one at a time, but you could have one for lunch and another for dinner. In order to create a complete meal out of the fourth category, you need to combine your preferred choice of protein with one or two vegetable dishes.

There are many reasons why we have chosen to eat this way. First, we have found that whenever we eat two proteins, such as shrimp and scallops, or beef and chicken, we come away feeling dissatisfied and irritated because we want to eat more—more volume and more variety.

The same principle applies to vegetables. If you eat a variety of vegetables every day, you begin to get bored with them because they always seem the same. But if you eat only one or two in a meal, you pay more attention to what you are preparing and how you prepare it, as well as the taste of it when you eat it.

In effect, eating this way becomes a form of meditation. You eat more slowly, you are mindful of what you are eating, and you are peaceful and satisfied afterward. Furthermore, you will appreciate that food again the next time you eat it, because that will be at least a week later. This not only makes food special to you but simplifies your life.

TABLE 9.2: HERBS AND SPICES

Allspice	Cinnamon	Lemon Mint	Saffron
Anise	Cloves	Lemon Thyme	Sage
Basil	Coriander	Marjoram	Salvia
Bay Leaf	Cumin	Mint	Savory
Caper	Curry	Mustard	Sesame Seeds
Caraway	Dill	Nutmeg	Sorrel
Cardamom	Fennel	Oregano	Spearmint
Cayenne Pepper	Garlic	Paprika	Tandori Masala
Celery	Garlic Chives	Parsley	Tarragon
Chervil	Ginger	Pepper	Thai Basil
Chicory	Juniper	Peppermint	Thyme
Chili	Lemon	Poppy Seeds	Turmeric
Chives	Lemon Balm	Rosemary	Vanilla
Cilantro	Lemon Basil	Safflower	Yarrow

TABLE 9.3: VEGETABLE CHOICES

First-Choice Vegetables (low in calories)			Second-Choice Vegetables (high in calories)
Artichokes	Chicory	Leeks	Avocado
Asparagus	Chinese Artichoke	Lettuce	Beets
Bamboo Shoot	Chives	Mushrooms	Carrots
Beet Tops	Cucumbers	Mustard Greens	Eggplant
Bell Peppers	Dandelion	Okra	Jerusalem Artichoke
Bok Choy	Dikon	Onions	Jicama
Broccoli	Endives	Radishes	Parsnips
Brussels Sprouts	Fennel	Shallots	Pumpkin
Cabbage	Garlic	Snow Peas	Squash
Cauliflower	Green Beans	Spinach	Turnips
Celeriak	Kale	Swiss Chard	Water Chestnuts
Celery	Kohlrabi	Tomatoes	Yacón
			Zucchini

Even when you are shopping for the food, you are not stuffing your basket with every item in the store, but are being selective and clear. On the other hand, when you have finished eating the food, you find that there is nothing to throw away, so you are not being wasteful. The way Americans eat today, it has been calculated that all the people in China could be fed for a year on what we throw away! Imagine how much money you could save if you kept eighty cents of every dollar you now spend on food.

There is one other benefit of simplifying your eating, and that is that it frees up time and energy for you to converse with other people. You are not focusing on what is on the menu, or on what you will eat next, but on the people you are with.

A friend of ours recently told us about what happened when he took his four-year-old son to a local toy store. The boy had a temper tantrum because he ran from one toy to the next, not spending much time with any, and then insisted on taking all of them home. Basically, he was overwhelmed by all the choices in front of him, and his four-year-old brain went crazy. That's what happens to us when we have too many kinds of food in front of us. We want to taste and eat all of them. And fast!

In the following pages, we will present food concepts and recipes that follow The Happy Body philosophy. As you eat these suggested meals, keep in mind that the purpose is for you to achieve and maintain your Happy Body.

CHAPTER 10

SOUPS & STEWS

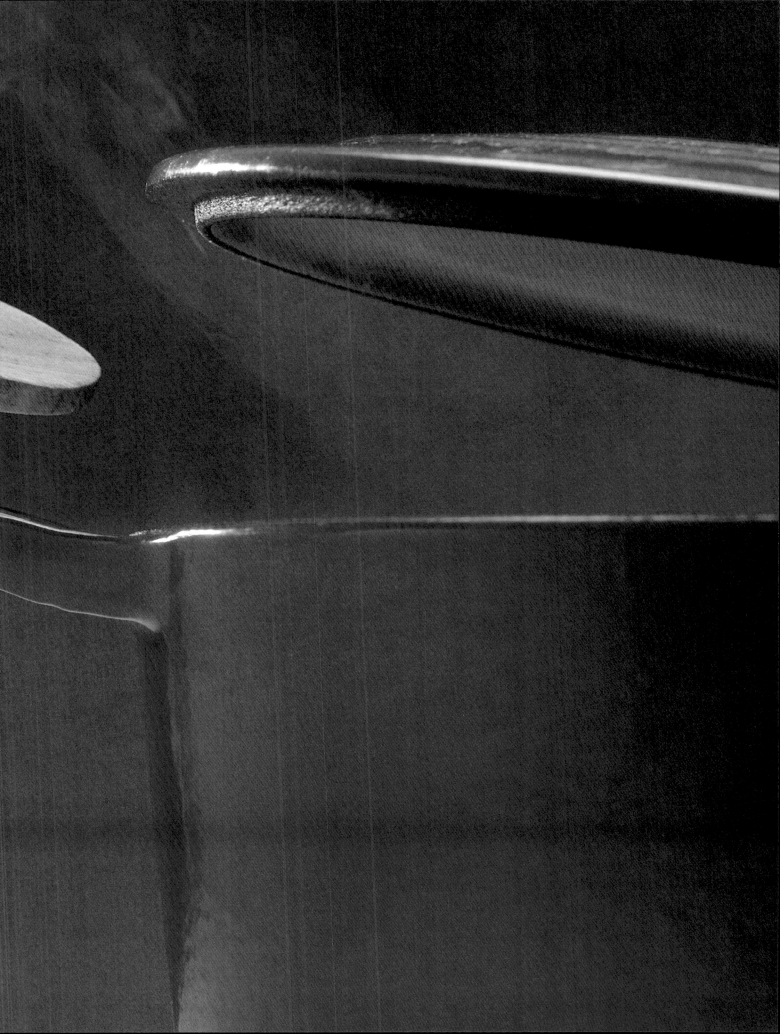

SOUPS AND STEWS

We like to eat freshly prepared, not reheated, food every day, looking for ways to eat at home with the least amount of time spent on cooking. With this in mind, we discovered that using a pressure cooker is one of the easiest and fastest ways to prepare great tasting soups and stews. What's the difference between soups and stews? The amount of liquid that's used. Soups are more liquid, whereas stews are more saucy. The amount of calories is the same in both.

There are many advantages to using a pressure cooker. The most important one is that it retains all the nutrients in the food, which also makes it tastier than food prepared in traditional ways. Furthermore, it is fast and efficient. A delicious fresh soup or stew can be prepared in only twenty minutes. Also, you can peel, cut, and pack fresh vegetables into containers on weekends, store them in the refrigerator or freezer, and use them during the week. As a last resort, if you don't have time for that, you can use frozen ingredients from your health food store.

Cooking with another person can make the process more fun. When we cook, we work as a team: one of us cleans and peels the vegetables, while the other one cuts them, and we enjoy each other's company at the same time.

As you put ingredients together, use your imagination. You can create a great tasting dish by unconventional ways of putting things together.

When we were a young couple and first started cooking together, we soon realized that we were making bland meals. Since we loved soups more than anything else, and Jerzy's mother, who was a great soup-maker, lived nearby, Jerzy asked her one day to teach him how to cook.

"Alright," she said, "let's start."

"Let me get a pencil and paper," Jerzy said.

"No pencils and no paper," his mom insisted. "We'll just see what's in the fridge."

"But how will I learn to do it again?"

"Every soup is different... and that's the whole fun of it."

So, she opened the refrigerator, and asked, "What vegetable do we have the most of?"

"Tomatoes," Jerzy said, "and they're ready to go."

"Then, we'll make tomato soup. First, we'll cut up some onions, parsley, carrots, leeks, and celery. Then we'll add water and throw in some chicken, beef, or beans. We have chicken, so we'll use chicken today."

"How much of each vegetable, Mamushka?"

"About the same amount of each."

"What if we don't have one of those vegetables?"

"We'll just use what we have. So long as we have any two of those ingredients, we'll be fine."

"But then we'll always be making a different soup. There won't be any consistency from one time to the next."

"That's the whole point. Every soup you make is unique. You can use five basic vegetables as half of any soup. Today, the other half will be tomatoes. And we'll always be sure to use salt and pepper to flavor our soups and stews. You can also add other spices and herbs."

For the next several weeks, Jerzy and his mom made soups with every possible combination of vegetables and proteins, and they were all delicious.

As you put ingredients together, use your imagination. You can create a great tasting dish by unconventional ways of putting things together.

Gaining Insight

Janelle L. White (40-year-old clinical psychologist)

For the past three years, my efforts to balance family and work had left my own self-care at the bottom of my To Do list. For many years I had prided myself on having an active lifestyle, including yoga, Pilates, and gym, that kept me healthy and fit, but in recent years I'd lost sight of how to make good exercise and food choices. With my 40th birthday around the corner, I certainly assumed age was going to work against any effort I might make to change my routine. That was until I read an article featuring Jerzy and Aniela Gregorek and their program The Happy Body. I was inspired by the positive results they reported with their 40-and-older clients. These were people who were dedicated to exercise and living healthy, like me, but often lacked reward from their efforts.

I began The Happy Body program, and within one month I experienced immediate results, which motivated me to keep going. In five months I have returned to a normal weight range and have become noticeably stronger and more flexible. What has kept me committed to the program has not only been the positive change to my body but also having access to Jerzy and Aniela's years of experience. You don't have to reinvent the wheel; their quantified plan clearly lays out what exercises to do and how to do them, and it keeps your food choices straightforward with minimal preparation. Because The Happy Body program requires patience (it does not happen overnight), you may discover ways that you end up sabotaging yourself. Having worked with individuals through the years, many who have struggled with being overweight, I know how important a consistent, nutritionally-balanced diet and active lifestyle are to good health. I also know that the reasons for not maintaining consistency may be very complicated. With the challenges that often occur when confronting and changing old habits, part of this journey really is about gaining insight into yourself.

Like many of Jerzy and Aniela's clients, my introduction to The Happy Body program began as a family commitment. I am so thankful that my husband began and will continue this journey with me, and that we can call Jerzy and Aniela friends. With The Happy Body program you have an opportunity to adopt a healthier way to live, gain a clearer understanding of your body and its potential, and learn what having a happy body really means.

Plan For Healthy Living

Lori Nawn (50-year-old corporate treasurer)

What do you call a woman who wears a bikini for the first time at the age of 50? A Happy Body and a happy soul!

When I met Jerzy and Aniela I was two months shy of my 50th birthday and had spent most of my life fighting my weight and my food demons. Sure, there were brief stretches of time when I would win the weight battle, but I invariably lost the war. I am 5'3" and my weight ranged from a low of 122 twenty years ago, to a high of 178 post-pregnancy. The vicious cycle of yo-yo dieting had become a way of life for me.

As my milestone birthday was approaching, I was becoming more and more frustrated with my inability to get my weight under control. An acquaintance mentioned The Happy Body and suggested that I get in touch with Jerzy. I checked out the website, made an appointment, and started immediately.

The great thing about The Happy Body program is that it addresses both food and exercise in a way that can be incorporated into any lifestyle. I didn't need a dedicated home gym or a personal chef to make this work. A few free weights, an exercise mat, and regular trips to the natural grocery store, and I was on my way! Jerzy and Aniela worked with me so that eating out and enjoying wine — the things I love — were not banished from my life.

To date, I've lost over 20% of my body weight in fat, gained 5% muscle, and have gone from wearing a tight size 8 to a comfortable size 2. I love my daily workouts — they are how I start my day. The Happy Body program isn't a diet, it's a reasonable plan for healthy living, and one that I hope to be following for the next 50 years of my life.

Cauliflower and Spinach Soup with Tarragon

Serves 2 to 4

Ingredients

2 tbsp of olive oil

1 cup of leeks, thinly sliced (white and pale green parts only)

1 lb. of cauliflower florets

1 turnip, peeled and cut into chunks

1 lb. of chicken or vegetable stock

1 lb. of baby spinach

2 tsp of fresh tarragon, minced

salt and pepper to taste

Preparation

- Warm the olive oil in a large saucepan.

- Add the leaks and sauté for 3 to 4 minutes until softened.

- Add the cauliflower, turnips, and stock.

- Bring to a simmer and cover.

- Cook until the vegetables are tender (about 20 minutes).

- Turn off the heat and stir in the spinach, which will wilt instantly.

- Purée the soup in a blender.

- Pour the soup into a clean saucepan and reheat.

- Season with tarragon, salt, and pepper.

Courtesy of Colette Cranston

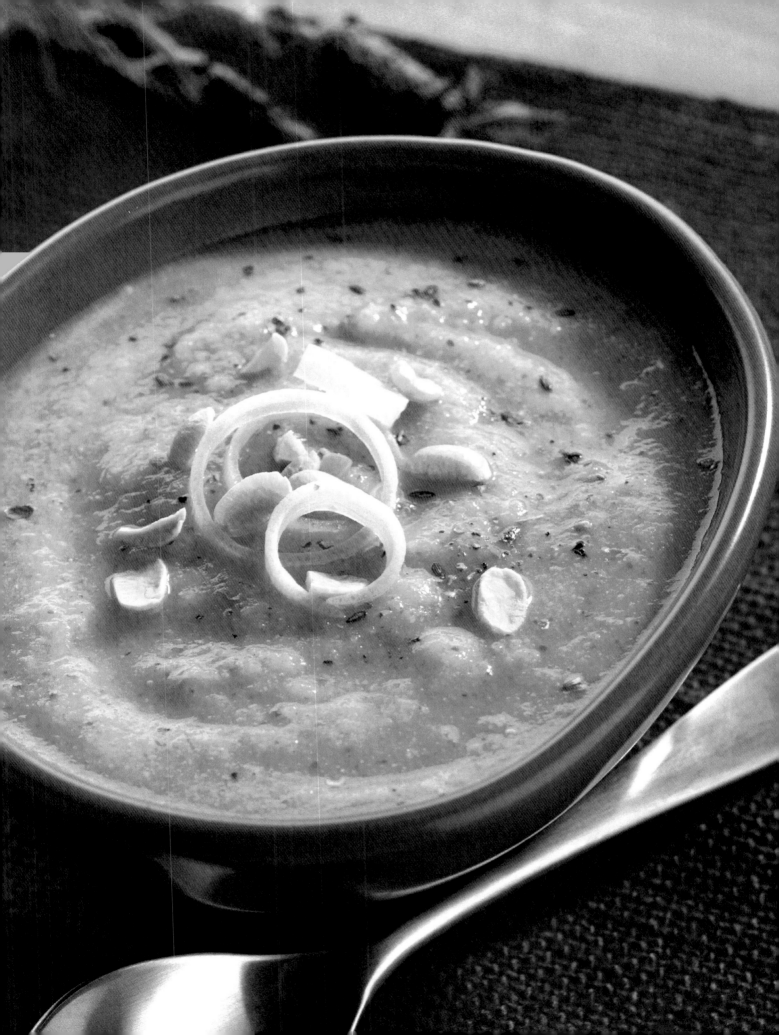

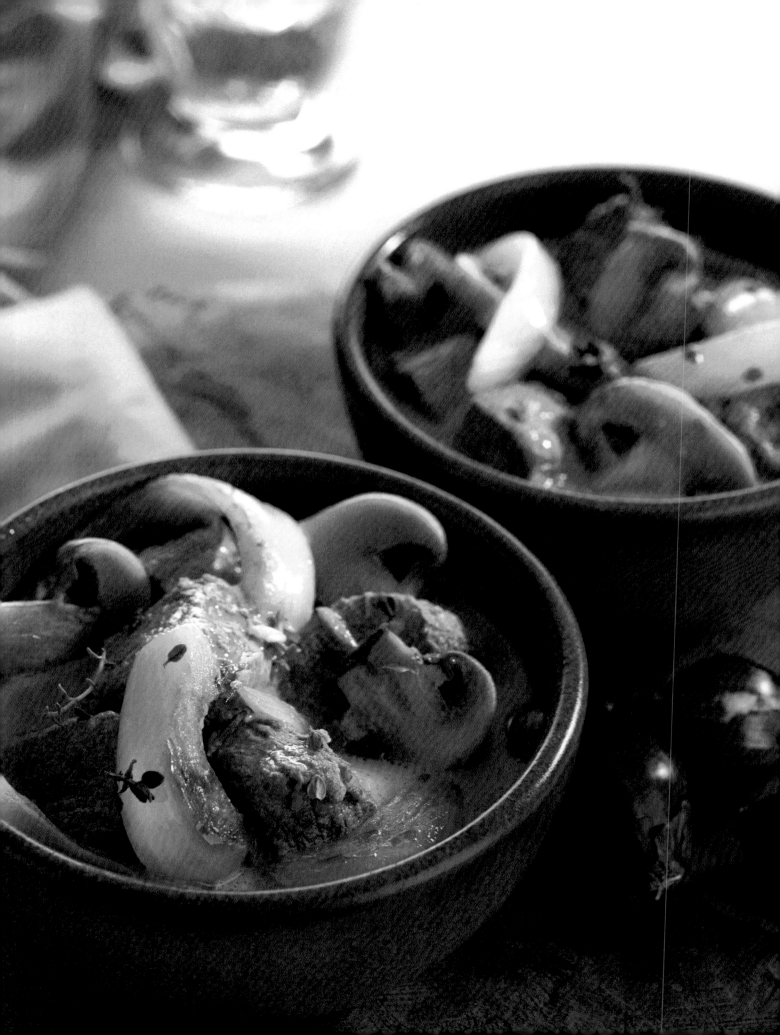

French Veal and Mushroom Stew

Serves 2 to 4

Ingredients

1 lb. veal, cut into small cubes

1 tbsp olive oil

2 cloves garlic, finely chopped

1 tsp Dijon mustard

2 tbsp fresh thyme, chopped

1 lb. mushroom, finely sliced

1 large onion, very finely chopped

1 tbsp lemon juice

1 tbsp fat-free sour cream

1 ½ cans chicken broth

salt and pepper to taste

Preparation

- Heat the olive oil in a medium-heavy iron casserole dish with the lid on.

- Add the veal and continue to cook over medium-high heat, stirring until each cube has lost its pink color.

- Add the garlic, thyme, mustard, salt, pepper, and chicken broth.

- Cover the casserole dish, place it in an oven set to 200° F, and bake for 3 to 4 hours. (The meat should be fork tender. The longer it is cooked, the more tender it becomes.)

- Sauté the onions with a bit of broth in a nonstick frying pan until they are slightly brown, and then let them cool.

- Sauté the mushrooms in the remaining broth until they are soft, and let them cool.

- When the veal reaches the desired tenderness, remove a cup of the gravy and pour it into a food processor with ½ of the sautéd mushrooms. Blend until smooth and place in the casserole dish.

- Add lemon juice and sour cream; stir.

- Add the other ½ of the mushroom and the onions.

- Return the dish to the oven for ½ hour more.

- Add salt and pepper to taste.

Courtesy of Christy Neidig

Chicken Vegetable Medley Soup

Serves 2 to 4

Ingredients

2 whole chicken breasts

2 zucchini, sliced

1 whole celery root, shredded

1 large leek, sliced

2 carrots, sliced

2 parsley roots, sliced

2 red bell peppers, sliced

1 cup of green beans, cut

1 large yellow onion, sliced

1 bunch of parsley, chopped (optional)

salt and pepper to taste

Preparation

- Put all ingredients in a pot and cover with water.
- Cook on the stove without bringing to a boil for 40 minutes.
- Take the chicken out of the pot, cut it into small pieces, and place it back into the pot.
- Add salt and pepper to taste.

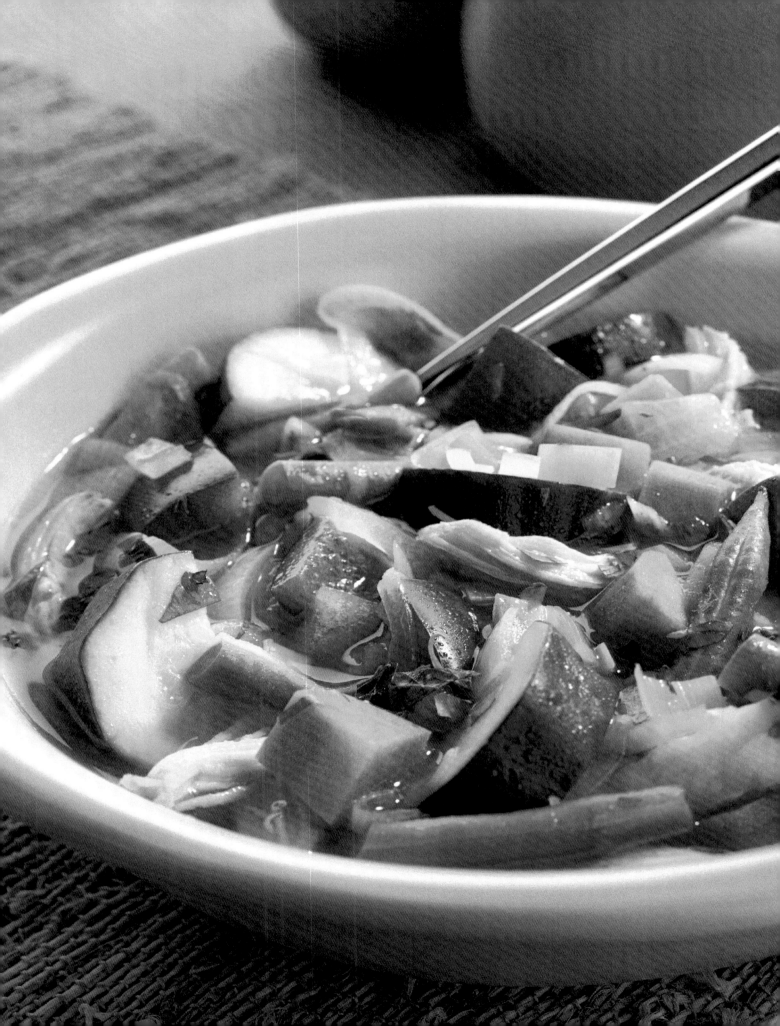

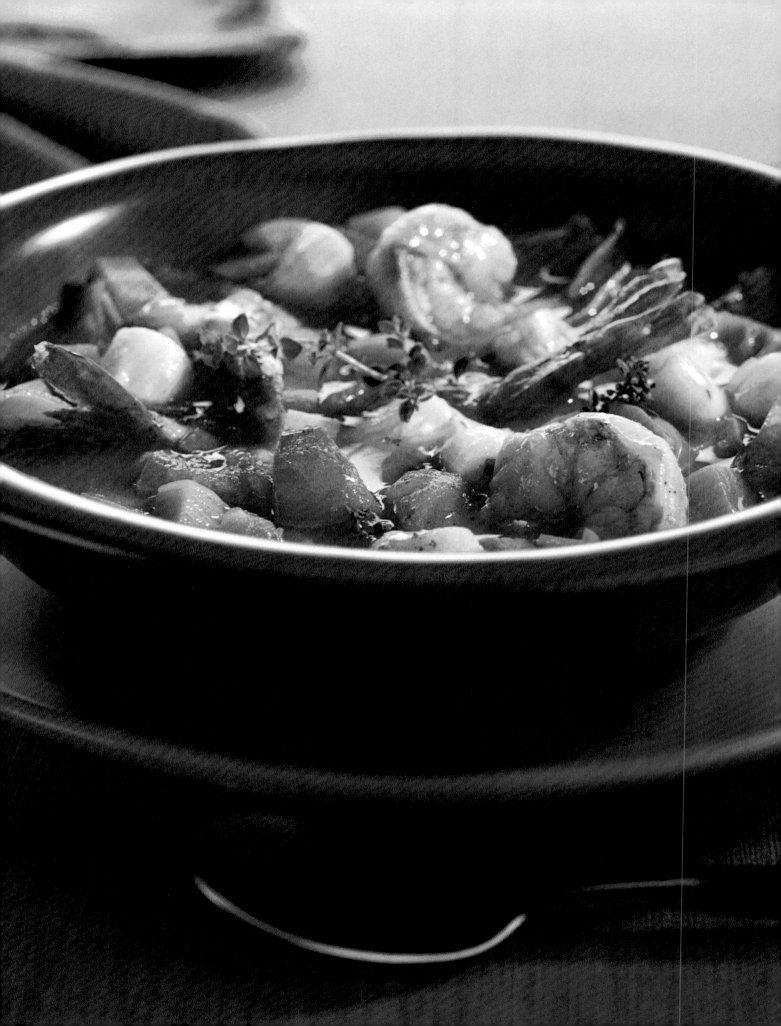

Seafood Stew

Serves 2 to 4

Ingredients

2 lb. of shrimp (or use a mix of shrimp, scallop, clams, and white fish)

1/2 lb. of sea scallop

4-6 leeks (white only), diced

10 cloves of garlic, minced

2 carrots, diced

5 cups of tomatoes (canned)

2 tsp of jalapeño pepper, seeded

2 cups of white wine

3 tbsp of olive oil

1 cup of fish stock (or water)

6 tsp of cilantro

2 tsp of cumin

1/2 tsp cayenne

1/2 tsp cinnamon

cilantro to top

Preparation

- Heat the olive oil over medium heat in a stockpot.
- Add the leeks and garlic
- Sauté until the ingredients are tender and translucent (approximately 10 minutes).
- Add the jalapeño, carrots, cumin, cayenne, and cinnamon.
- Decrease the heat to medium low and cook until the carrots are almost tender.
- Add the tomatoes, wine, and fish stock.
- Bring to a boil and then lower the heat to medium for 5 minutes.
- Stir in the shrimp or other seefood.
- Cook until the seafood stew is just cooked through.
- Top with cilantro leaves and serve.

Courtesy of Peggy Dow

Spicy Beef Soup

Serves 2 to 4

Ingredients

1 lb. lean beef, cubed

2 celery sticks, chopped

2 carrots, sliced

1 leek root, sliced

1 green bell pepper, chopped

1 small yellow onion, minced

2 tbsp olive oil

1 tsp smoked red paprika

1 tsp cumin

2 bay leaves

$\frac{1}{3}$ cup dill pickles, chopped

2 tbsp fresh parsley, chopped

salt and pepper

Preparation

- Heat the olive oil in a large saucepan.
- Sauté the meat and onion together.
- When the meat is browned and the onion is soft, transfer them to a soup pot.
- Add all the vegetables to the pot.
- Cover all the ingredients with water and add two more cups of water.
- Add the paprika, cumin, bay leaves, salt, and pepper.
- Simmer for 20 minutes.
- Garnish with the dill pickles and parsley.
- Serve hot.

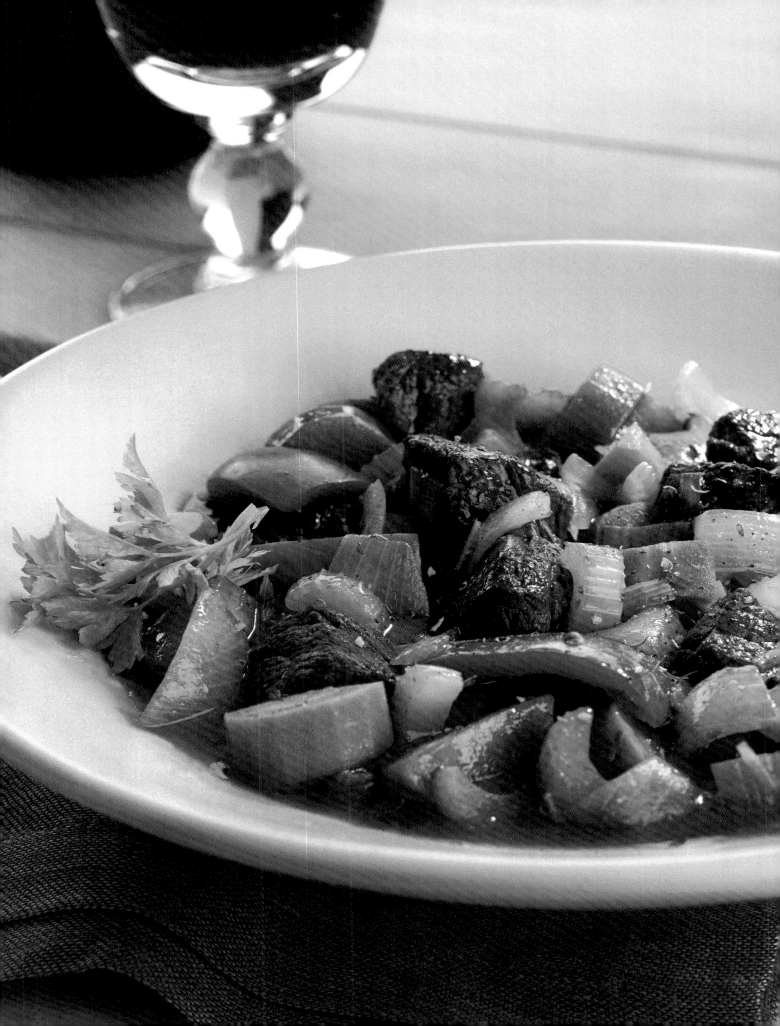

My Blood Work is Perfect

Samantha Dinsmore (58-year-old housewife)

I am a fifty-eight-year-old woman who always fought to gain even one pound during the first three decades of my life. Yes, fought to *gain*, not lose. I could enjoy potatoes, rice, pasta, french fries, milk shakes, and my favorite desserts without any thought and without gaining any weight. At twenty-nine I was below 100 pounds even though I ate anything and everything that I wanted without guilt or weight gain.

Everything changed in my late-thirties. I went through early menopause and realized that my metabolism had changed even though my eating habits had not. I started to gain a pound at a time, which led to five pounds then ten pounds.

Like many of my female friends, in my forties all I had to do was think about dessert and I gained weight. My body's ability to ward off weight seemed to have changed overnight. I was leading an active lifestyle, but since exercise had never really been a part of my daily routine, I honestly hadn't given it much priority.

In my fifties, the weight gain increased. I was now up to almost 140 pounds. My 5'5" frame was literally uncomfortable. My knees and my neck ached, and I had now developed *osteopenia*, a condition characterized by low bone mineral density.

On the side of vanity my clothes had been replaced for the next size up all too often. The positive was that I knew how to dress and could disguise my rolls and lumps beautifully. The negative was that I was only fooling those on the outside: I knew that my own personal health and well-being were suffering. So, I joined a local workout facility and worked with a trainer three days a week. I was feeling a little stronger, but my body was not cooperating. I wasn't shedding the pounds.

It was Christmas when I realized that it was finally time to start taking care of myself. I had raised two daughters and devoted all of my time to them. Now it was time to make myself the priority.

A friend referred me to Jerzy and Aniela. When I went to my initial meeting, I went home wondering how I was going to live on The Happy Body regime. That first week I even told my husband, with tears in my eyes, that there was no way I could do this. At the end of that week, when I went for my first weigh in, I had actually lost weight. By the end of the first month I lost ten pounds! I was now committed.

The Happy Body program has taught me the importance of how nutrition and exercise work together. You can't have success unless you have both of these components working as a team. They also taught me how food works: starch turns

[CONTINUED ON NEXT PAGE]

into sugar, which turns into unnecessary and unhealthy calories. These were relationships that I had never truly understood before. They are the essentials to living a happy life and to having a happy body.

Over the years I have fluctuated at times, but I always come back to the basics. I have seen so many positive changes in my health and well being, including the fact that my knees and neck no longer hurt. As a matter of fact, I can't remember the last time that anything hurt. My internist reports on my annual physical report that my blood work is "perfect," my *osteopenia* has also improved, and I have never felt better.

CHAPTER 11

SALADS

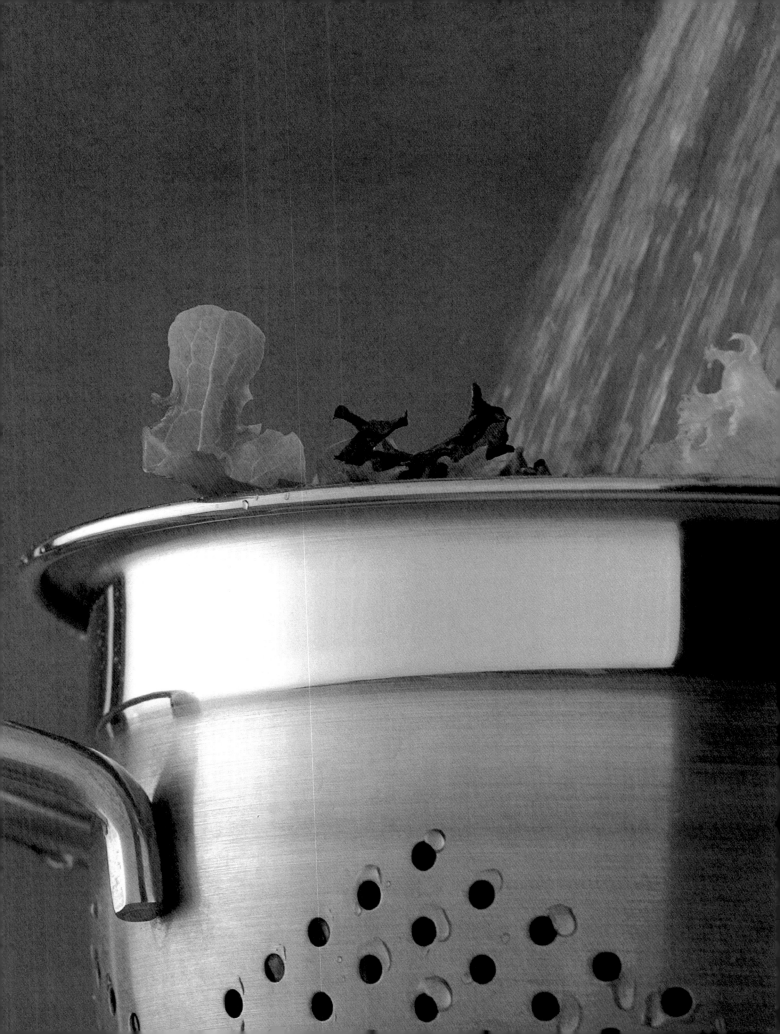

SALADS

J ust as soups are especially satisfying in the cold months, salads are especially enjoyable in the warm months. There is nothing better on a hot day than nourishing and cooling off your body with fresh vegetables. They contain water, fiber, vitamins, minerals, and enzymes, and, when you add protein to them, they can stabilize your energy throughout the long day.

Ideally, you should eat at least one pound of vegetables every day for every hundred pounds of your Ideal Body Weight. When you make a salad, the ratio of vegetables to protein and fat should be 70/20/10 by calories for men, and 70/17/13 for women. The trouble is that most people make salads that are 10 percent vegetables, 20 percent protein, and 70 percent fat. The effect of that, because of the lack of roughage and volume, is constipation. The protein should be as lean as possible, such as in chicken breasts, turkey breasts, top sirloin, fish, seafood, or egg whites. All of these ingredients except egg whites contain fat. Therefore, when you make salads with egg whites, you should add some oil or nuts to bring the fat content up to the desired 10 or 13 percent.

It's hard to go wrong with salads if the vegetables are organically grown and fresh. We buy all of our vegetables at the local farmers' market or natural food store, where you can find a wide variety of tasty and exotic produce. For example, we have found tomatoes that taste like pineapples; cucumbers that taste like lemons, and mint that tastes like chocolate. You can also find uncommon herbs and spices, such as smoked garlic.

In salads, as with all of our food suggestions, experiment with different combinations of ingredients.

When You Are Ready, The Teacher Appears

Terry Oliver (53-year-old business woman)

Meeting Jerzy and Aniela changed my whole life. I was overweight, in pain, depressed, and heading down a path toward chronic illness. Life was overwhelming. In spite of all the walking I had done, I had gained twenty-five pounds over the previous seven years. I had severe pain in my joints, especially in my shoulders, elbows, ankles, little finger, and hips. I was also having severe hot flashes and rosacea on my cheeks. At fifty three, I felt old and discouraged.

At the time, I thought my diet was reasonably good because I ate lots of vegetables and fruit. But I also had wheat bread at every meal and desserts with every lunch and dinner. I knew intuitively that someone must know how to help me, but there are so many people giving advice on diet and exercise. Who could I trust?

I turned first to books for the answer. One of them taught me about the depleting nature of the typical American diet and how it leads to chronic disease. Eating excessive amounts of refined sugar is especially destructive to the body so I gave up my desserts and immediately felt much better. I didn't know at that time that health is not solely about sugar consumption but about having a balanced diet.

Everyone knows that diet is essential to long-term health and well being, but the book made everything too complicated. Hours of exercise a day and complicated meal plans were not for me. I needed to find a simpler way.

Five days after I gave up desserts, I ran into an old friend I'd not seen in a long time. She looked fantastic — twenty years younger — and was bubbling with enthusiasm for life.

I asked, "What have you done to change so dramatically?"

"The Happy Body!" she responded, and told me about Jerzy and Aniela's program. I called them right away and made an appointment for that very evening.

Over tea, Jerzy and Aniela explained their program to me, which combines a balanced diet with non-exhaustive exercises and relaxation techniques. The diet was easy to understand and follow and would simplify my eating habits and my grocery shopping.

Once I started the program, my joint pain vanished. It was a miracle! I also found that my hot flashes were less intense, and the rosacea started to clear up. In fact, my whole body was changing, I was losing body fat and building muscle at the same time. In six months I gained ten pounds of muscle while losing 40 pounds of fat. My total weight went down from 162 to 132. Now I'm more attractive, stronger, and more flexible. My life has become exciting again!

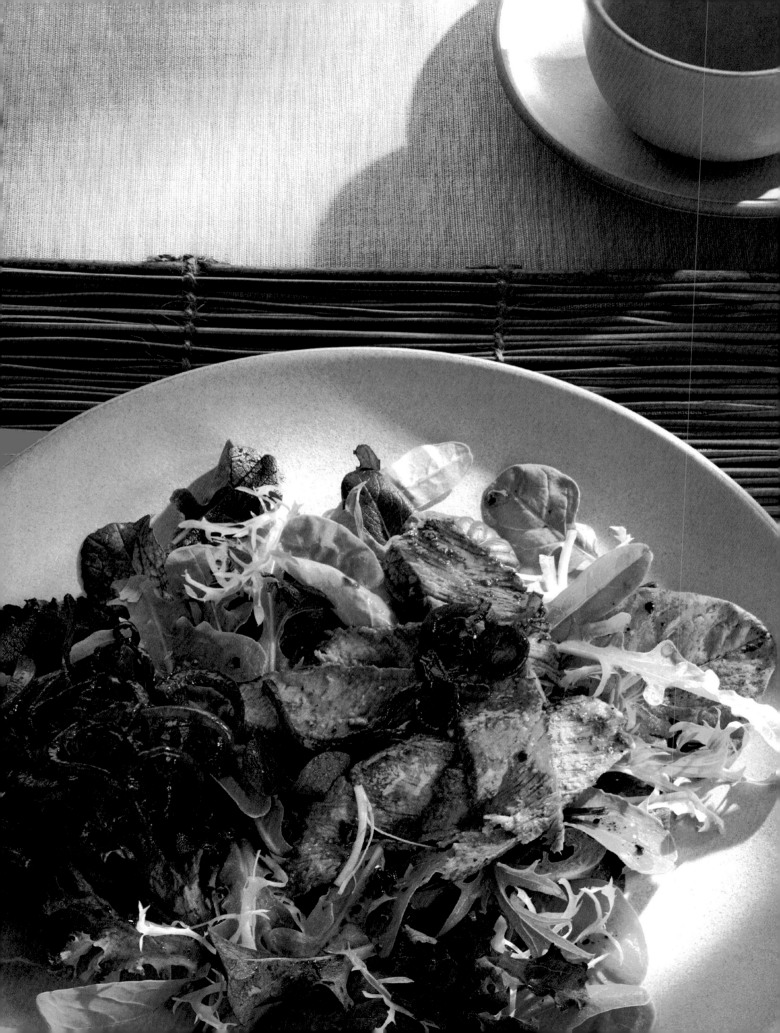

Balsamic Onion Salad with Steak

Serves 2 to 4

Ingredients

mixed baby greens

2 large red onions, sliced

$\frac{1}{3}$ cup of red balsamic vinegar

2 tbsp of virgin olive oil

leftover steak (6 ounces per serving)

salt

Preparation

- Preheat oven to 350º F.

- On a baking sheet, use your hands to stir thinly sliced onions, balsamic vinegar, olive oil, and salt.

- Bake for 10 minutes, then cool.

- Place the greens, onions, and steak in a large salad bowl, toss lightly, and serve.

Courtesy of Judy Finch

Beef Lettuce Wraps

Serves 2 to 4

Ingredients

1 lb. of beef, thinly sliced

1 head of lettuce with large leaves for wrapping

1 carrot, julienned

1 cucumber, julienned

1 cup of asparagus, steamed

¹⁄₂ cup of enoki mushrooms

¹⁄₂ cup of sprouts

Marinade:

2 tbsp of low sodium soy sauce

2 tbsp of balsamic vinegar

1 tsp of toasted sesame oil

2 tsp of Stevia (or other type of sweetener)

Preparation

- Combine all the marinade ingredients in a bowl.

- Place the beef slices and the marinade in a large Ziploc bag.

- Marinate for 3 hours, turning the bag over every half hour.

- Pan fry or broil the marinated beef without using additional oil.

- Wrap the beef and vegetables with the lettuce leaves and serve.

Courtesy of Helen Werdegar

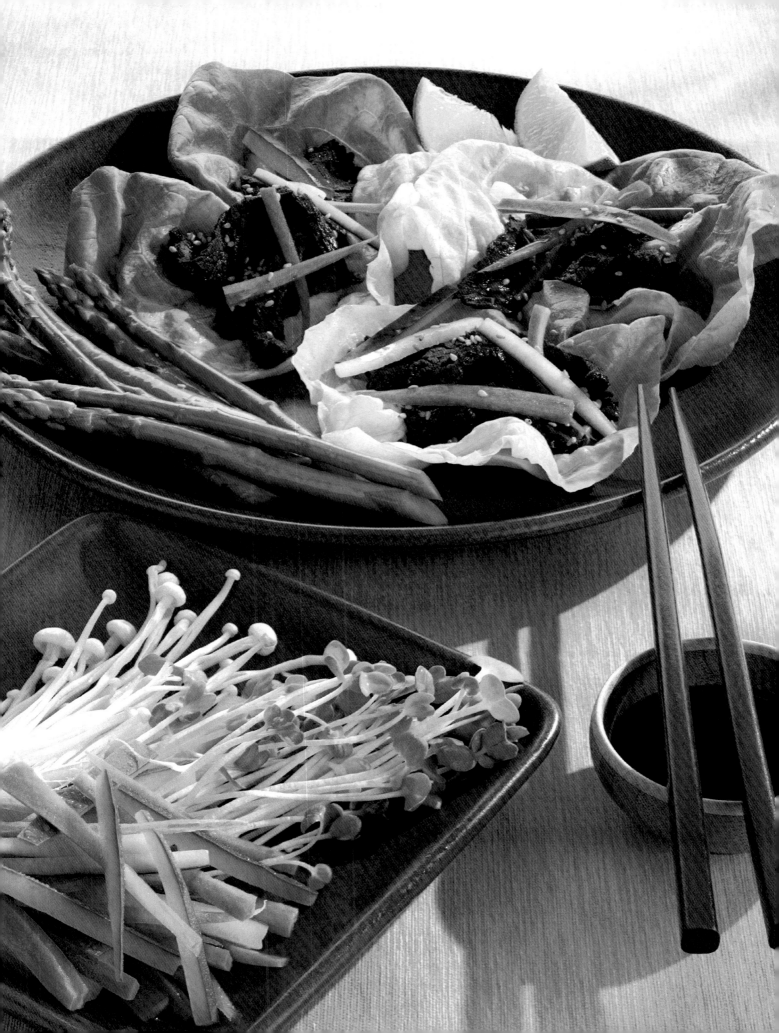

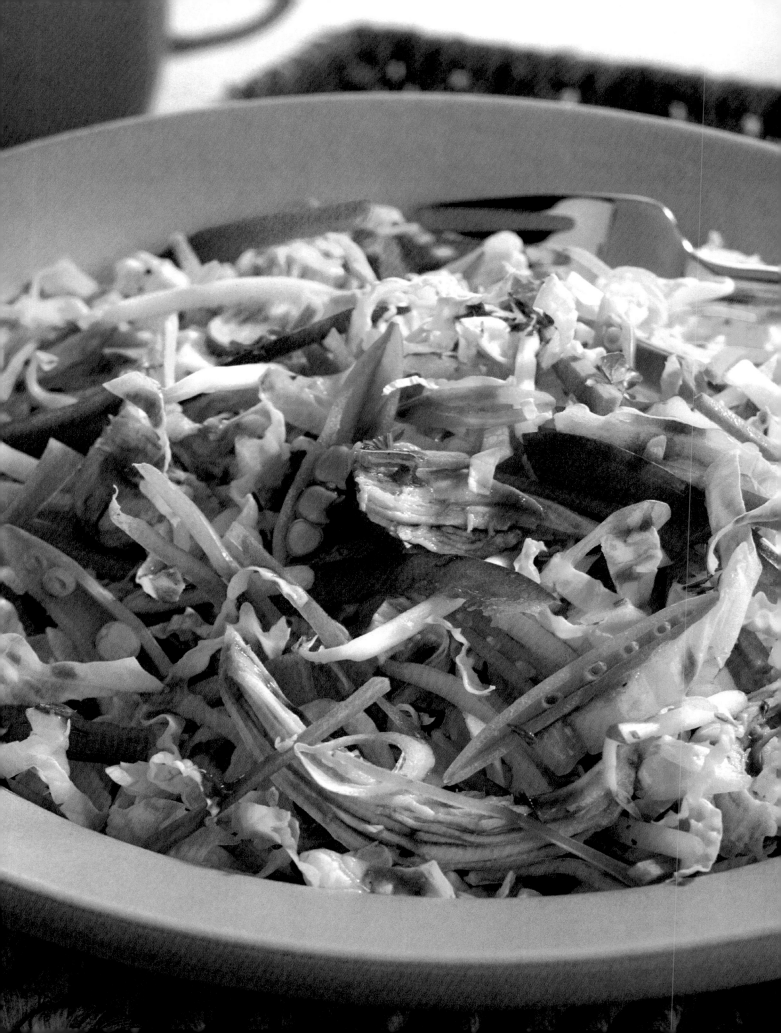

Hoisin Chicken Salad

Serves 2 to 4

Ingredients

2 boneless, skinless chicken breasts (1 lb.)

4 tsp of peanut oil

1/3 cup of rice vinegar

3 tbsp of hoisin sauce

1 1/2 tbsp of soy sauce

1 tbsp of fresh ginger, grated

1 carrot, peeled and grated

1 medium-sized head of Napa cabbage, sliced thin crosswise

1 large red bell pepper, stemmed, seeded, and sliced thin

1 cup of bean sprouts

2 scallions, sliced thin

1/2 cup of snap peas

1 tbsp of fresh cilantro, minced

salt and pepper

Preparation

- Pat the chicken dry with paper towels, then season generously with salt and pepper.

- Heat 1 tbsp of oil in a large nonstick skillet over medium-high heat.

- Place the chicken in the skillet and cook until browned on the first side (about 5 minutes).

- Flip the chicken over, add 1/3 cup of water, and reduce heat to medium-low.

- Cover the skillet and continue to cook until the thickest part of the breast is no longer pink and registers 165º F on an instant-read thermometer (about 5 to7 minutes).

- Transfer the chicken to a plate and cover with plastic wrap.

- Poke a few vent holes in the wrap and refrigerate while preparing the other ingredients.

- Mix the rice vinegar, the remaining 3 tsp of peanut oil, the hoisin sauce, the soy sauce, and the ginger together for the dressing.

- Shred the cold chicken into bite-size pieces.

- Combine the shredded chicken with the cabbage, carrot, bell pepper, bean sprouts, scallions, snap peas, and cilantro.

- Add the dressing and toss well to mix.

Courtesy of Peggy Dalal

Mexican Chicken Cups

Serves 2 to 4

Ingredients

2 whole chicken breasts, cooked (1 lb.)

1 head of iceberg lettuce leaves

1 large tomato, chopped

1 avocado, sliced

1 bunch of green onions, chopped

5 black olives, sliced

$\frac{1}{2}$ cup of nonfat cheese (preferably cheddar or Monterey Jack), grated

1 tbsp of taco seasoning

salsa or hot sauce

Preparation

- Cut the chicken breast into chunks.
- Add the taco seasoning.
- Place the chicken in individual lettuce cups.
- Top with the tomatoes, avocado, onions, olives, and cheese.
- Add salsa or hot sauce to taste.

Courtesy of Judy Kiel

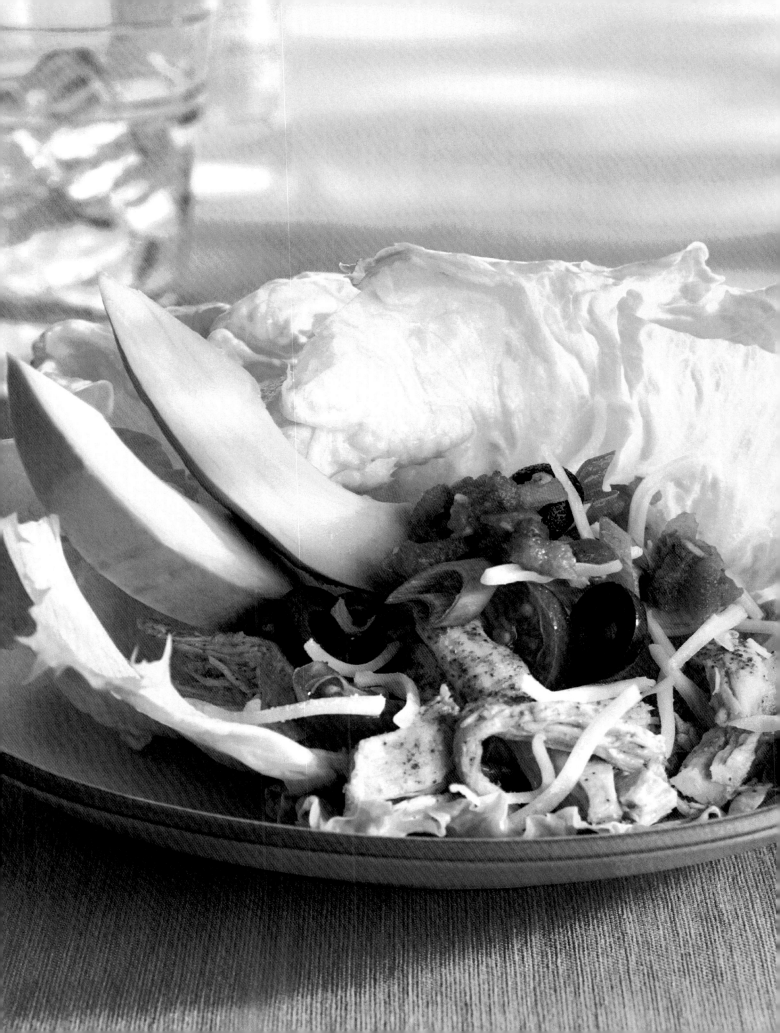

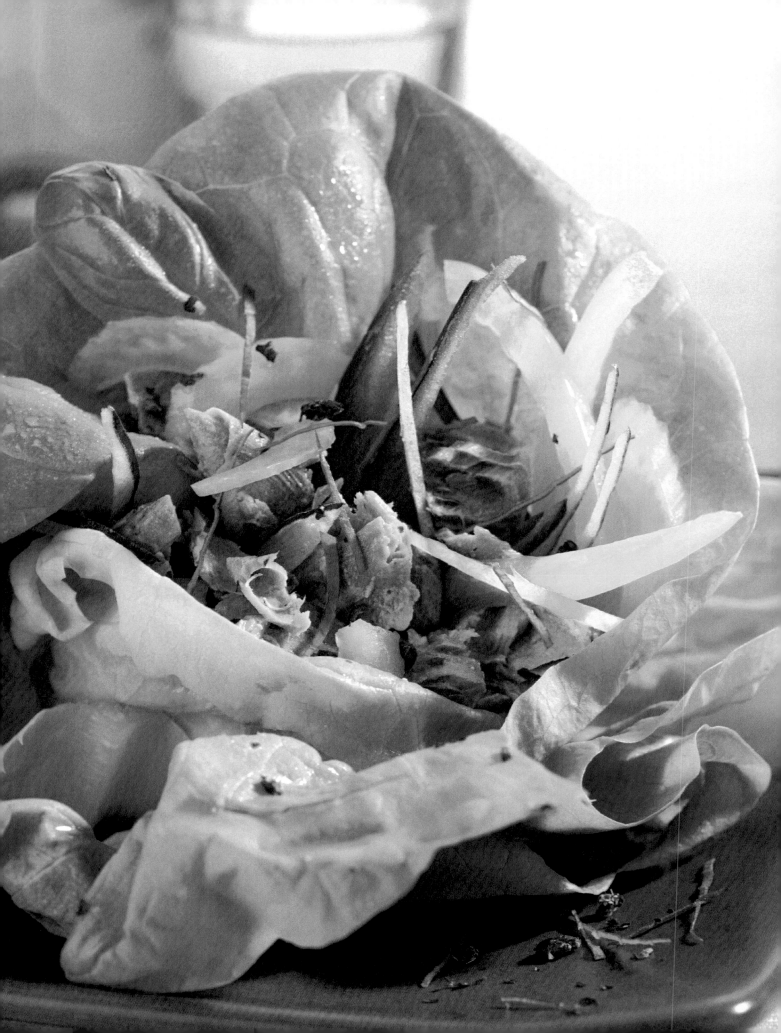

Salmon Cups

Serves 2 to 4

Ingredients

1 head of butter lettuce leaves

1 lb. of boneless Alaskan wild salmon

2 celery stalks, minced

$\frac{1}{2}$ red onion, minced

1 red bell pepper, minced

1 yellow bell pepper, minced

Salad Dressing

$\frac{1}{4}$ cup of extra virgin olive oil

4 tbsp of fresh lemon juice

4 tbsp of fresh basil

2 cloves of garlic

salt

Preparation

- Bake the salmon at 350º F for 20 minutes.
- Arrange the lettuce leaves on a dish.
- Fill the lettuce leaves with the minced vegetables.
- Add chunks of salmon on top.
- Make the dressing by mixing all the ingredients in a blender.
- Pour the dressing on top of the salmon.

Courtesy of Barbara Stefik

CHAPTER 12

EGG WHITE DISHES

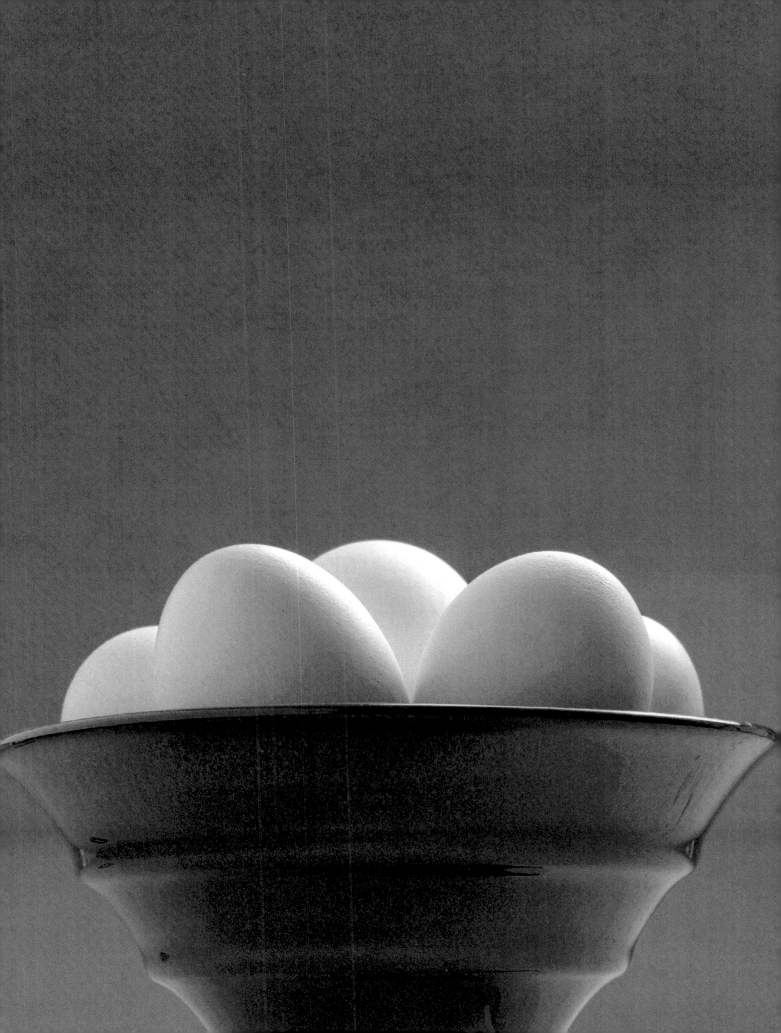

EGG WHITE DISHES

Most people think of eggs as perfect food. Although an egg white, which contains 16 calories, is almost pure protein, the yolk contains 56 calories and is mostly saturated fat. So if you eat eggs, you should only eat the whites, especially while you are losing fat. For example, if you make an omelet out of six egg whites and a pound of vegetables, your omelet will be 200 calories. However, if you make it out of whole eggs it will be 550 calories.

But not all eggs are equally healthy because most of them are produced by chickens that are given hormones and antibiotics. The healthiest eggs come from chickens that run free and are not fed any chemicals.

Egg whites can be prepared as a snack with bread or vegetables, or they can be added to a main dish, such as a salad or soup. The simplest and easiest way to prepare eggs is to hard-boil them and discard the yolks. The next easiest method is to separate the raw yolks and whites, and then scramble the whites or turn them into omelets. (If you are concerned about waste, you can buy egg whites alone in health food stores, or if you like to garden, you can use the yolks for compost.)

Again, feel free to play and experiment with these recipes. Eating egg whites does not have to be boring; it's what you eat with them that makes them flavorful. Here are some recipes for making egg white dishes. You can alter the proportions or spices as you wish, so long as you stay within The Happy Body guidelines.

Winning the Sugar War

Helen Scheffler (56-year-old interior decorator)

I started The Happy Body program expecting to fail. After all, I'm not an athlete, and I've been addicted to sugar forever. Although I had been thin most of my life, I was resigned to my ever-increasing menopausal spread.

Fortunately, Jerzy and Aniela know more than I do about health and fitness, so thanks to their diet, exercise, and meditation plan, I stopped craving sugar after only two days.

It's now three years later, and I've not only kept off the pounds but lost what Jerzy calls my "winter coat of blubber."

I'm still not athletic, but the exercise plan is not difficult — it only takes a small part of my day — and I can tell the difference in the way I feel and move. I intend to follow the diet and exercise regimen for a long time to come.

Mushroom Soufflé

Serves 4 to 8

Ingredients

24 egg whites

5 zucchinis

1 yellow onion

1 lb. of white mushrooms

1 lb. of crimini mushrooms

2 tbsp of olive oil

parsley (optional)

salt and pepper

Preparation

- Preheat oven to 425° F.
- Shred the zucchinis, mushrooms, and onion in a food processor.
- Place the mixture in a bowl.
- Add the egg whites.
- Season with salt and pepper and stir.
- Grease a casserole pan with olive oil.
- Place the mixture in the pan and bake for 1 hour or until brown.

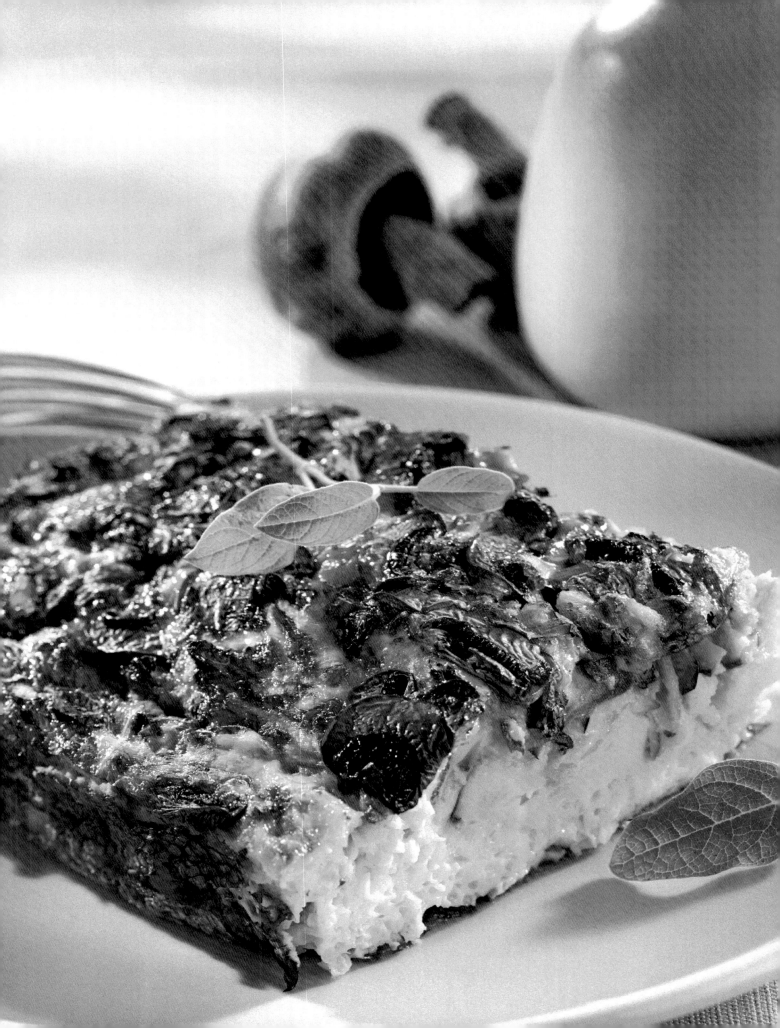

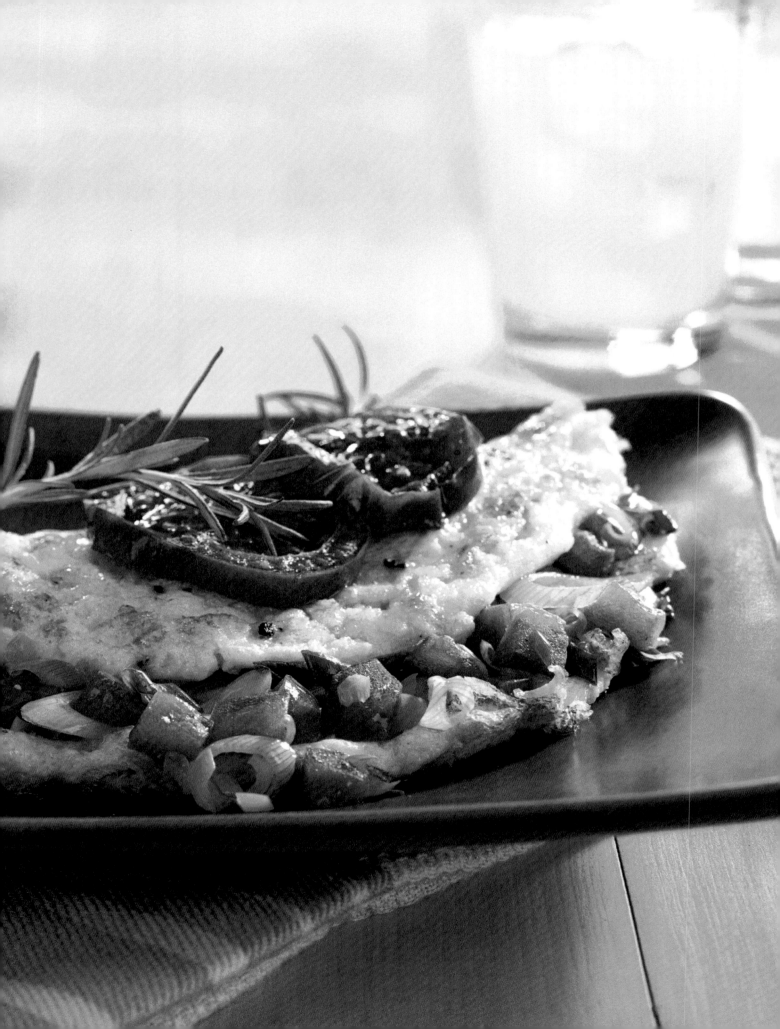

Tomato, Onion & Basil Omelet

Serves 1 to 2

Ingredients

6 egg whites

1 beef tomato, diced

1 bunch of green onions

2 tbsp of fresh basil, chopped

3 tsp of olive oil

¼ cup of nonfat milk

salt and pepper

Preparation

• Coat a nonstick skillet with a thin layer of olive oil.

• Heat the skillet.

• Sauté the onions until they are soft.

• Add the diced tomato and cook for another minute.

• Sprinkle in the basil and put the mixture aside on a plate.

• Place the milk and egg whites in a bowl.

• Whisk the mixture until the consistency is even.

• Season with salt and pepper.

• Recoat the skillet with a thin layer of olive oil.

• Reheat the skillet.

• Pour the egg white mixture into the skillet and spread the contents evenly by tilting the skillet.

• Loosen the mixture from the skillet with a spatula and cook it on a low flame until the egg whites set.

• Place the onion and tomato mixture on the left half of the egg white pancake and fold the right half of the pancake over it.

• Cook the omelet for 2 minutes.

• Slide the omelet off the skillet onto a plate and serve it hot.

Tomato Stuffed with Egg Whites and Salmon Paste

Serves 1 to 2

Ingredients

2 egg whites, hard-boiled and chopped

⅓ cup of smoked or poached wild salmon

1 large beef tomato

1 cucumber, sliced

1 tsp of parsley, chopped

1 tsp of dill, chopped

mustard

salt and pepper

Preparation

- Cut the top off the tomato, put the top aside, and spoon out the inside of the tomato.

- Prepare the paste by placing the salmon, parsley, dill, mustard, salt, and pepper in a blender.

- Mix the paste with the egg whites in a bowl.

- Stuff the mixture into the tomato and cover it with the tomato top.

- Serve with slices of cucumber.

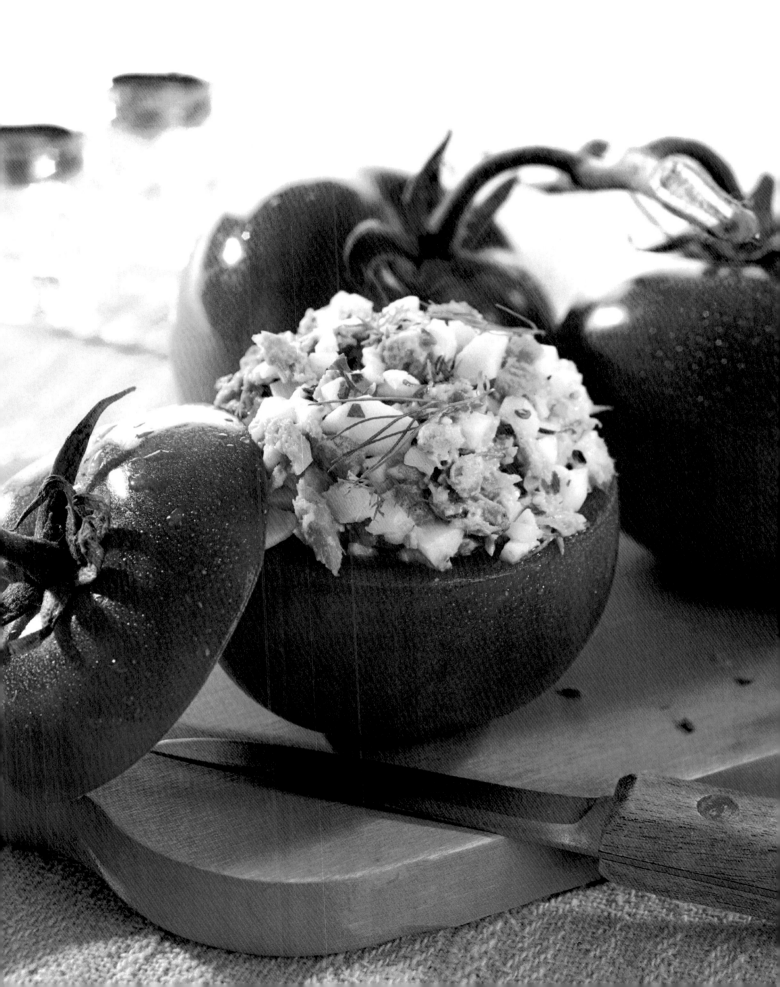

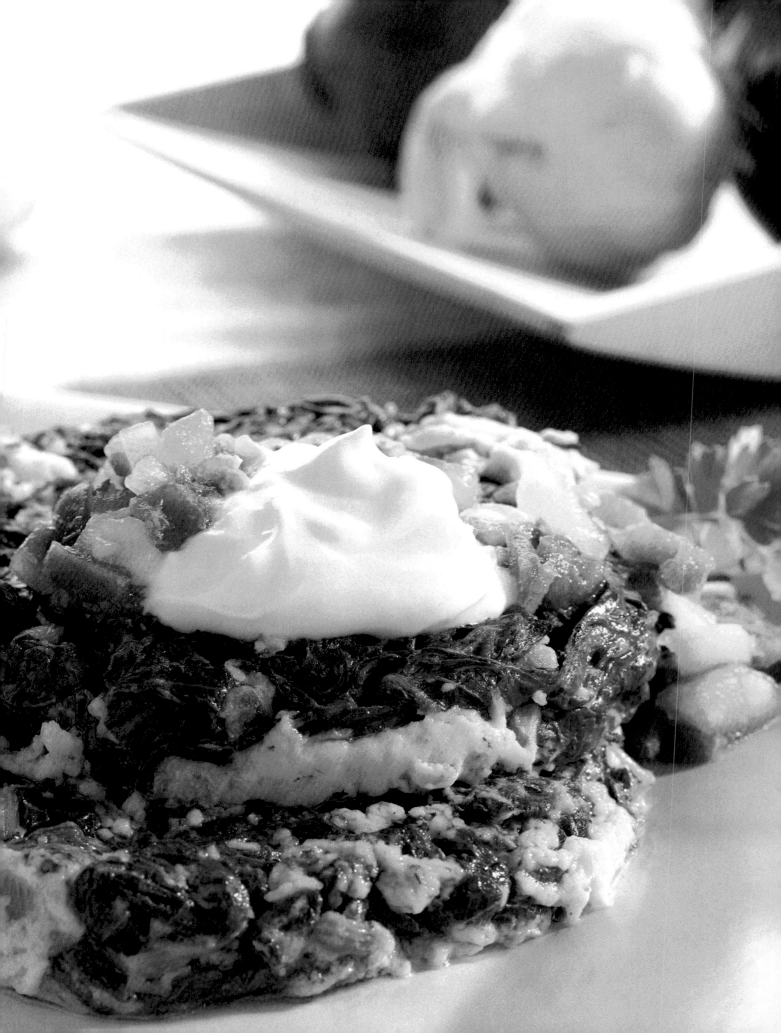

Spinach Pancakes

Serves 2 to 4

Ingredients

2 lbs of fresh spinach

12 egg whites

1 cup mozzarella cheese, fat-free, shredded

1 small onion, finely chopped

1 bunch of fresh parsley, chopped

½ cup of Greek yogurt

½ cup of salsa

olive oil

salt and pepper

Preparation

- Steam the spinach for 1 minute and let cool.
- Heat 2 tbsp of the olive oil in a nonstick skillet.
- Sauté the onion.
- Mix the spinach, onion, parsley, egg whites, and cheese in a large bowl.
- Add salt and pepper to taste.
- Coat the skillet with a thin layer of olive oil to prevent the pancakes from sticking.
- Reheat the skillet.
- With a tablespoon, ladle out pancake-size portions into the skillet.
- Cook the pancakes on both sides.
- When the pancakes are ready, put them on a plate.
- Top each one with 1 tsp of Greek yogurt and 1 tsp of salsa.

Egg White Frittata with Smoked Salmon

Serves 2 to 4

Ingredients

12 egg whites

7 oz. of smoked salmon, shredded

4 Roma tomatoes, cut into wedges

4 cups of fresh spinach, chopped

4 tbsp of chives

2 tbsp of dill

4 tbsp of olive oil

2 cloves of garlic, minced

salt and pepper

Preparation

• Heat 2 tbsp of olive oil in a frying pan.

• Sauté the garlic and salmon in the pan for 3 minutes.

• Add the tomatoes and spinach and sauté for another minute or until the spinach is wilted.

• Remove from the heat.

• Add the chives and the dill.

• Season with salt and pepper.

• Heat the oven to 350º F.

• Pour 2 tbsp of olive oil into an oven-proof nonstick skillet.

• Pour the egg whites into the skillet.

• Spoon the salmon mixture into the center of the skillet.

• Swirl the mixture into the egg whites.

• Bake until the egg whites in the center are puffed and cooked (approximately 12 minutes).

• Serve hot or cold.

Courtesy of Lorna Basso

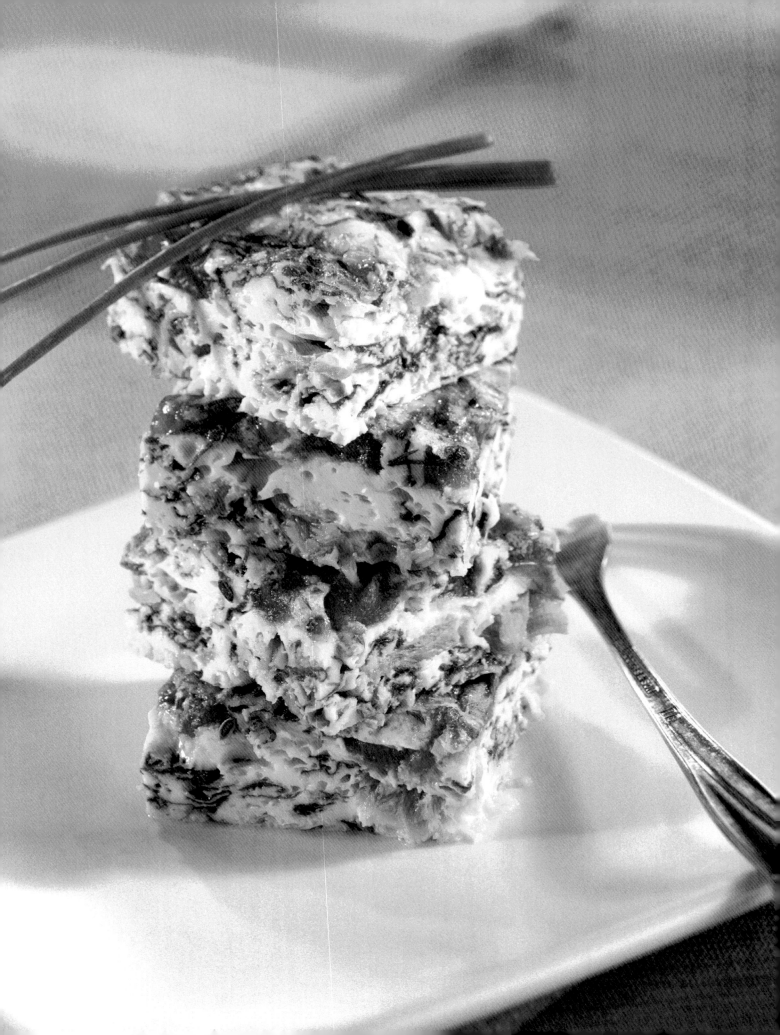

Living My Life to the Fullest

Ritu Ghumman (37-year-old veterinarian)

O nce my journey with The Happy Body program began, I never looked back. I am a working mom of three children aged 7, 6, and 1. The Happy Body has changed my way of living, eating, and thinking, and it has taught me how to make the right choices.

Initially, when I was trying to find a weight loss program that would help me shed the last 15 pounds after the birth of my second child, I came across an article about The Happy Body program in a magazine. It was very inspiring. I had been with personal trainers for the past 3 years, working out three times a week. I had pretty much tried all the weight loss programs that are available where I live, but my last 15 pounds just stayed on me. I had to give this program a try.

I remember meeting Jerzy and Aniela for the first time in their home and listening to what they had to say about The Happy Body. The best part for me was when they took me to the meditation room. Meditation as part of a weight loss program? That completely took me by surprise. I soon realized, though, that The Happy Body is not just about losing weight but about changing your lifestyle. It sculpts your body and your mind. It improves you physically and mentally.

In just 6 weeks, I lost 12 pounds on The Happy Body program. I was ecstatic. I just couldn't believe it!

But, three months into the program I got pregnant with my third child. I tend to gain a lot of weight with my pregnancies, and this time I ended up gaining 60 pounds. I came back to Aniela and Jerzy 4 months after delivery, and I have lost all of the weight. I feel great, and I look great — not just because I have lost weight, but I now have learned how to live my life to the fullest through this program.

I Am a Better Golfer

Lauren Buchanan (17 year-old student)

I started The Happy Body program at the beginning of the summer. I wanted to lose fat and gain muscle. I never dreamed that an unexpected bonus was that it would make me a better golfer.

I have been playing golf seriously for four years. Before I began The Happy Body Program, I was hitting my drives on average between 190 and 200 yards. After just six months working with Jerzy and Aniela, most of my drives are between 210 and 230 yards, and I can occasionally hit drives up to 260 yards.

Talk about a confidence booster! Not only is my golf game better, but so is my balance and posture. I used to slump over when I walked, but with new exercises that Jerzy gave me, I now walk tall.

I had a hard time at first believing that a half hour of simple weight-bearing exercise and a simple-to-follow food program could do so much for my body. Since I began the program, I have lost 15 pounds of fat and gained 5 pounds of muscle. My overall weight will go up as I keep working to gain muscle.

My friends ask me if The Happy Body program is a diet. It most certainly is not. The Happy Body program is a way of life. I eat five times a day, and I'm never hungry. In fact, I'm often too full to eat the next meal. By volume I eat a lot, but I keep my fat consumption to a minimum, which has improved the quality of my skin. Although I have a very busy day as a high school senior and captain of the varsity golf team, I have no problem fitting the half hour of exercises into my schedule.

Last year, whenever I got up for school, I was exhausted and rundown. I still stay up late at night working on homework, but the meditation aspect of The Happy Body program and the teas and other meditative exercises that Aniela suggests have really helped strengthen my mental health. I am calm, less stressed out, and much more energized.

I am now stronger on and off the golf course, and I have newfound vigor for life. I owe this all to Jerzy and Aniela.

CHAPTER 13

FREE-CHOICE DINNERS

FREE-CHOICE DINNERS

Many of our clients asked us if we could hold dinners from time to time to share healthy recipes with each other. We thought that was a fantastic idea, so we decided to invite them to a potluck dinner once a month. The only rules were that they had to bring meals that were delicious and compatible with The Happy Body philosophy. Also, the recipes had to be original. They could have been handed down for generations in families, or they could have been invented yesterday, but they could not be from cookbooks. Some people brought complete meals, but others brought dishes that only contained meat, fish, or vegetables. As our guests began to mix these in different combinations, we realized that they were creating complete meals out of side dishes in original ways.

As the months passed by, our clients began to tell us that they were inspired by our potluck dinners to eat free-choice meals at home. One of our clients, Katie, told us how this style of eating had changed her family over time without even trying.

"When I first started The Happy Body program," she said, "Jerzy asked me to teach my family mutual respect at the dinner table. So I sat down with my husband, Al, and my kids, and told them that I would be eating differently than before, but I would still cook everything they wanted to eat. That would be my respect for them. And their respect for me would be not to offer me their food, which they knew I didn't want anymore. But it was hard for me to look at and smell those bowls of buttered corn or pasta alfredo, which still made me salivate. I would finish my steak and green beans, and they would go on eating and eating until there wasn't a scrap left. Then, after one of your potlucks, I got the idea to serve my dinners the same way you do. At first, Al and the kids were irritated that they had to get up and go to the kitchen all the time to get their own food. Nevertheless, they kept loading up, as always, with the same old things. The only difference was that there was a lot of running back and forth from the kitchen to the dining room. But it was much easier for me to eat my way when I wasn't tempted by those bowls of macaroni and cheese, which sat in the other room. After a month or so, I noticed that my family was making fewer trips to the kitchen, and they were even leaving some food—and it was always the high calorie carbohydrates, like rice, potatoes, corn, and pasta. So I started making meals with less of those things and more vegetables. Then I started introducing Happy Body recipes, such as mashed cauliflower instead of mashed potatoes. The first time I put mashed cauliflower on the counter, Al looked puzzled, as if to say, 'What's this?' After he tasted it, however, he said, 'Not too bad.' But my four-year-old daughter said, 'I really, really like this, Mommy!' I've been making free-choice dinners like this for five months now. The trips to the kitchen have stopped, so we spend more time with each other at the table, talking and laughing. My grocery bill is a third of what it used to be, and I cook a third of the amount of food that I used to cook. And the best part is that my husband and kids have lost weight, look healthier, and are more relaxed."

"I've been making free-choice dinners like this for five months now. My grocery bill is a third of what it used to be, and I cook a third of the amount of food that I used to cook. And the best part is that my husband and kids have lost weight, look healthier, and are more relaxed."

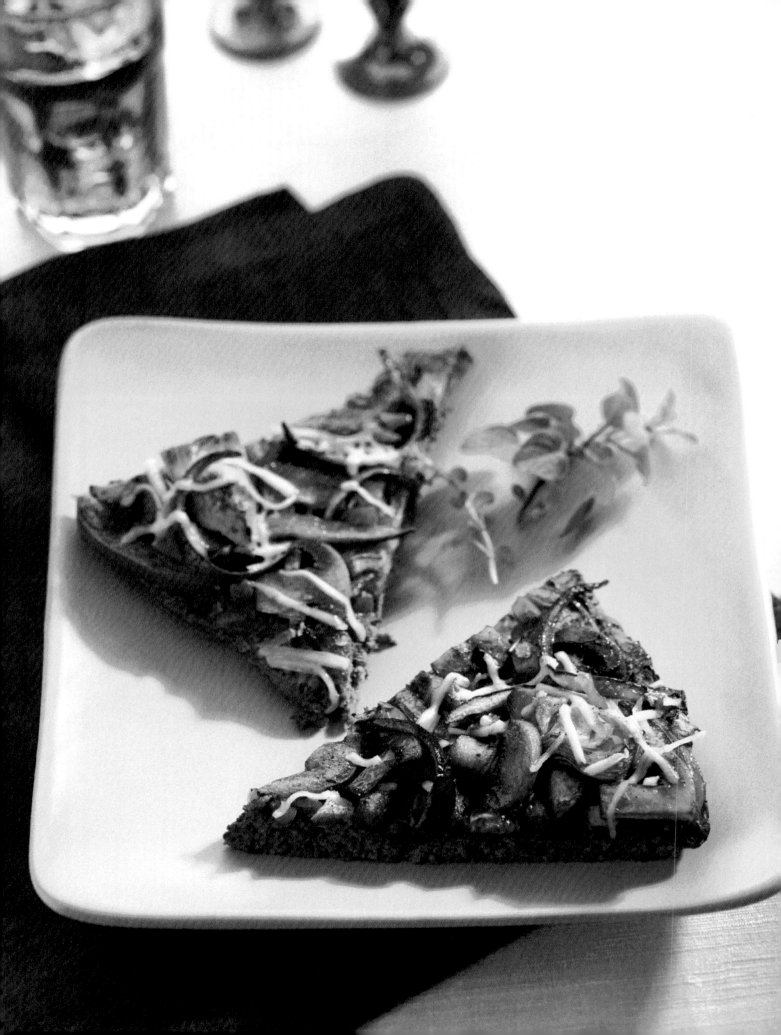

Beef-Crust Pizza

Serves 2 to 4

Ingredients

1 pound of beef, ground

½ cup of artichokes, frozen or marinated

1 large beefsteak tomato, sliced

½ cup of mushrooms, sliced

1 bell pepper, chopped

1 small red onion, chopped

4 cloves of garlic, minced

⅓ cup of non-fat cheese, grated

¼ cup of tomato sauce

2 tablespoons of olive oil

½ tsp of oregano

½ tsp of sweet basil

½ tsp of paprika

garlic salt

pepper

Preparation

- Season the meat with garlic salt and pepper.

- Knead the meat.

- Smear olive oil on the bottom of an oven dish.

- Lay out the seasoned meat in the oven dish the way dough would be for regular pizza.

- Spread the tomato sauce on the meat crust.

- In the following order, place the mushrooms, red onion, bell pepper, artichokes, tomato, garlic, oregano, basil, paprika, and pepper on top of the meat.

- Sprinkle the grated cheese on top.

- Bake at 350° F to taste (40 to 60 minutes).

Barbequed Flank Steak

Serves 2 to 4

Ingredients

2 lbs of flank steak

$\frac{1}{3}$ cup of soy sauce

2 tsp of apple juice

5 garlic cloves, minced

2 tsp of parsley, chopped

2 tsp of thyme, chopped

2 tsp of basil, chopped

pepper

Preparation

- Mix all the ingredients except the steak in a bowl.
- Coat the steak with this marinade.
- Let the steak marinate overnight.
- Barbecue.

Courtesy of Peggy Dow

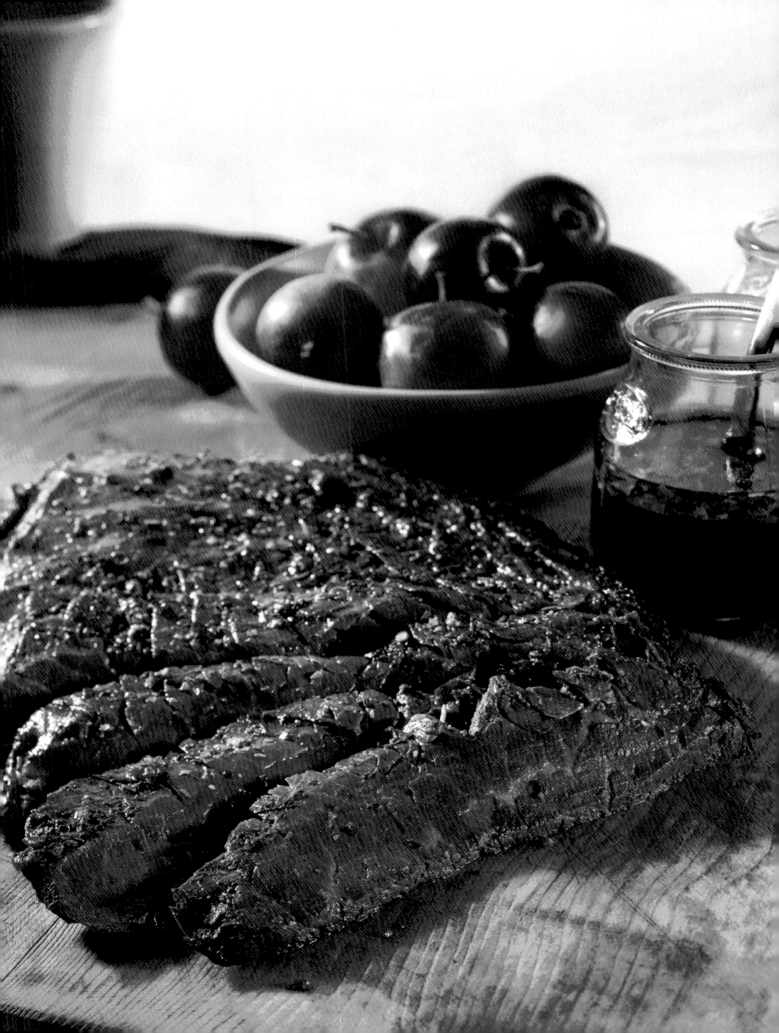

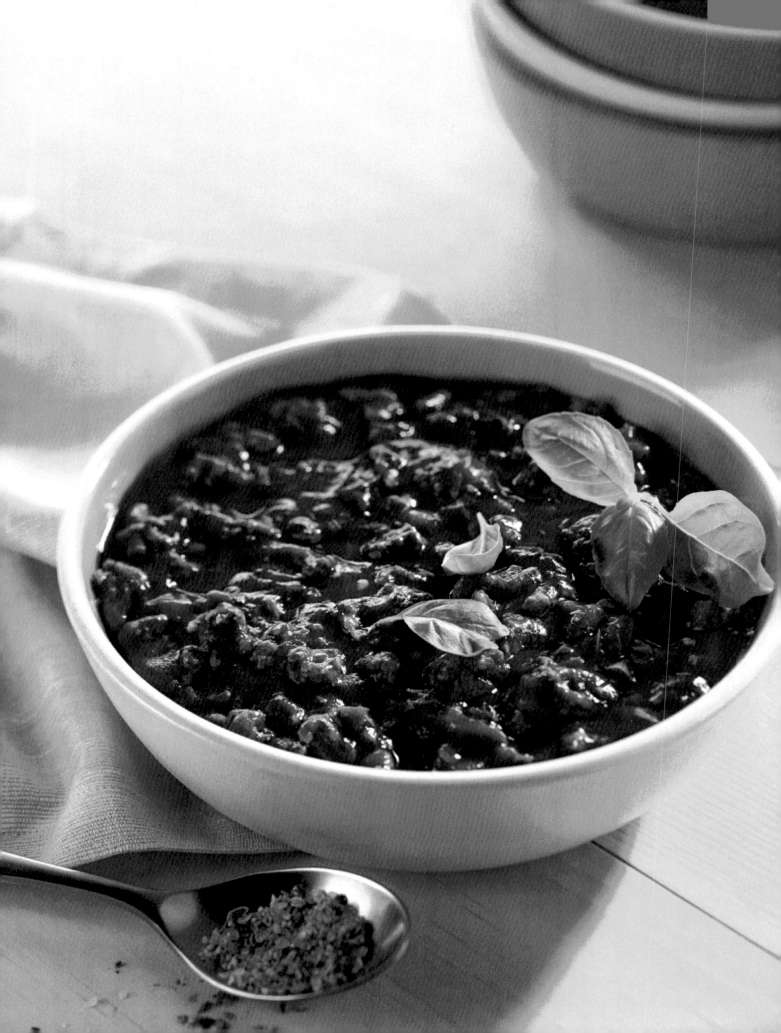

Ground Turkey Breast with Sauce

Serves 2 to 4

Ingredients

1 lb. of ground turkey breast

2 26-oz. bottles of tomato sauce

5 cloves of garlic, crushed

Italian herbs

basil, fresh

red pepper

black pepper

1/3 cup of red or white wine

salt

Preparation

- Place the ground turkey breast in an open pot and cook on high heat until the meat turns white.

- Add the tomato sauce, stir, and simmer for 3 minutes.

- Add the wine, stir, and continue simmering for 5 minutes.

- Add all the seasonings except the basil. Stir and continue simmering for 2 minutes.

- Add the basil, stir, and remove the pot from the heat.

Courtesy of Judy Kiel

Moroccan Chicken on a Skewer

Serves 3 to 6

Ingredients

6 boneless and skinless chicken breasts (2 lbs)

1 tbsp of olive oil

2 cloves of garlic, crushed

¹⁄₃ cup of lemon juice

¹⁄₂ tbsp of cumin

¹⁄₂ tbsp of coriander

salt and pepper

Preparation

- Cut the chicken into 1" cubes.
- Sprinkle the cubes with the other ingredients in a small bowl.
- Toss to blend.
- Refrigerate the chicken for 3 hours.
- Coat a grill with a nonstick cooking spray.
- Put the chicken cubes on skewers.
- Place the skewers on the hot grill for 6 to 7 minutes, turning once.
- Serve with Tzarziki Sauce (Greek yogurt dip).

Courtesy of Christy Neidig

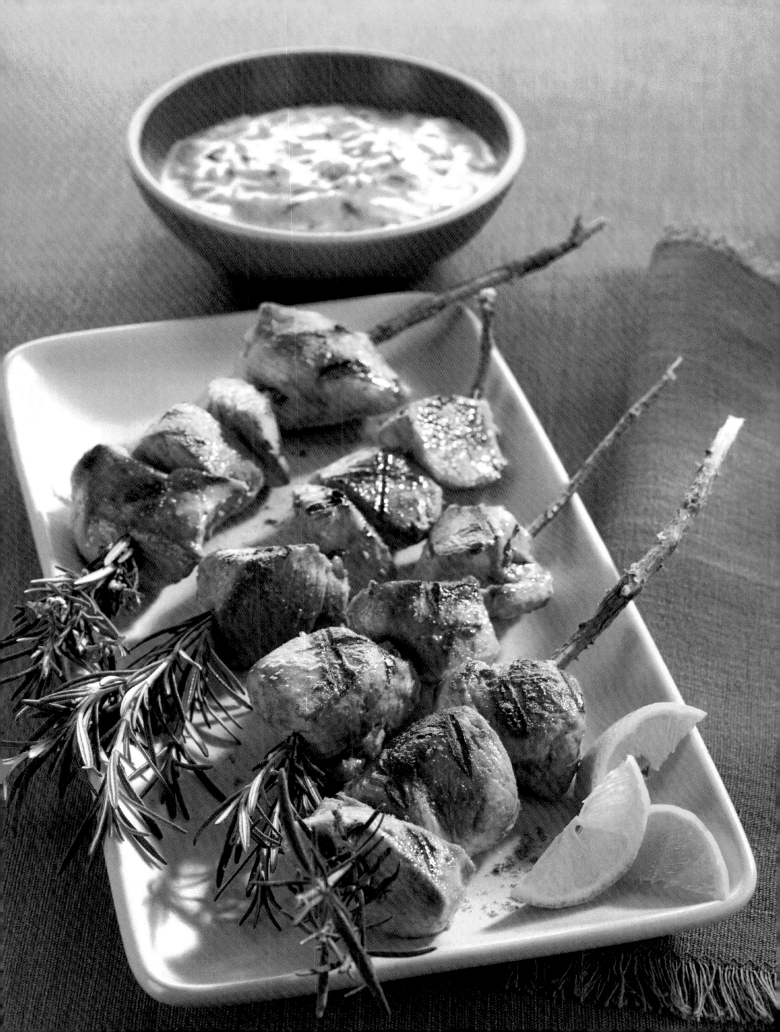

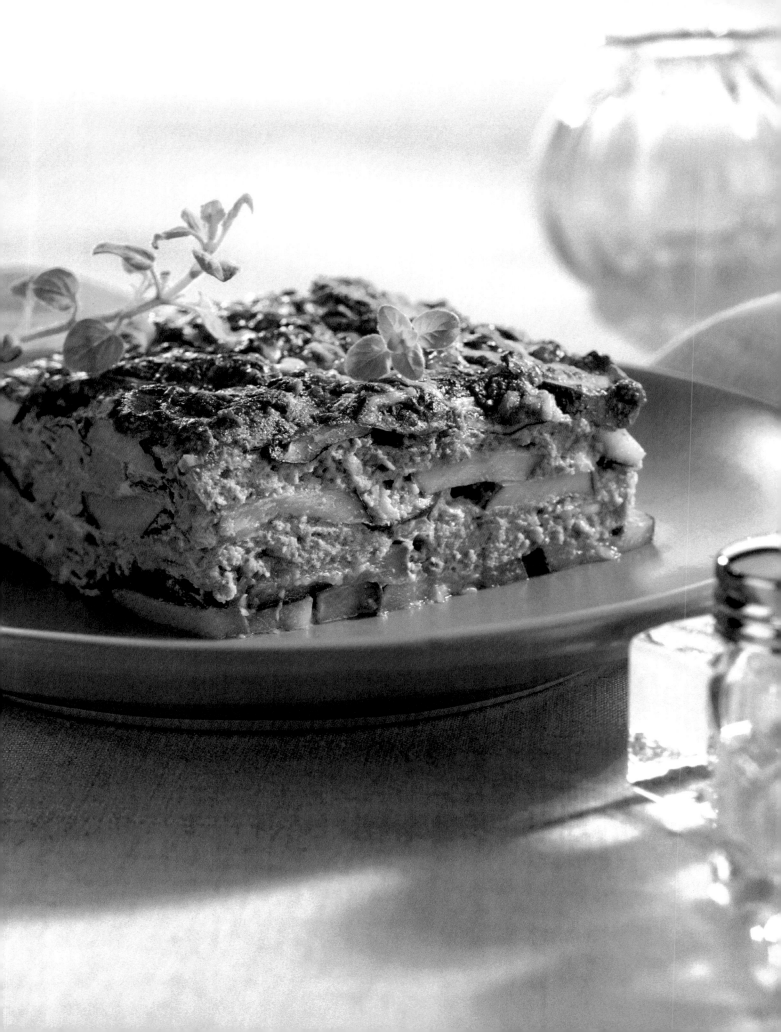

Turkey Lasagna Without Pasta

Serves 3 to 6

Ingredients

1 ½ lbs of turkey breast, ground

1 lb. of mushrooms

2 green bell peppers

1 lb. of spinach, finely chopped

1 yellow onion

5 cloves of garlic

16 oz. of nonfat cottage cheese

4 tbsp of low-fat parmesan cheese or soy cheese

5 egg whites

1 can of tomato sauce

4 large zucchini (to substitute for pasta)

4 tbsp of olive oil

garlic salt

pepper

Preparation

- Wash the zucchini and remove both ends.

- Cut the zucchini into thin diagonal slices.

- Smear the olive oil on top and sprinkle on garlic salt.

- Place the slices on a hot grill and cook on both sides until they are soft.

- Put the slices aside on a plate to cool.

- Blend the mushrooms, onion, garlic, and bell peppers in a food processor.

- Place the mixture in a bowl and add the turkey, spinach, cottage cheese, and egg whites.

- Add pepper and gently stir all the ingredients.

- Cover the bottom of a baking dish with the grilled zucchini.

- Spread a thin layer of the turkey mix on top of the zucchini.

- Cover the turkey mix with more zucchini.

- You can stop at 3 layers or create more, as you wish.

- Pour the tomato sauce on top.

- Sprinkle on the parmesan or soy cheese.

- Bake at 350º F for 45 minutes.

- Let it cool before you serve it because it gets really hot.

Lemon-Spicy Shrimp

Serves 2 to 4

Ingredients

1 lb. of shrimp

juice from 1 whole lemon

1 tsp of ground masala

1 tsp of chili oil

1 tsp of red pepper flakes

2 garlic coves

Preparation

• Marinate for 2–3 hours.

• Drain the marinade.

• Sauté in a pan on high heat until the shrimp turns from gray to pink-white.

Courtesy of Peggy Dow

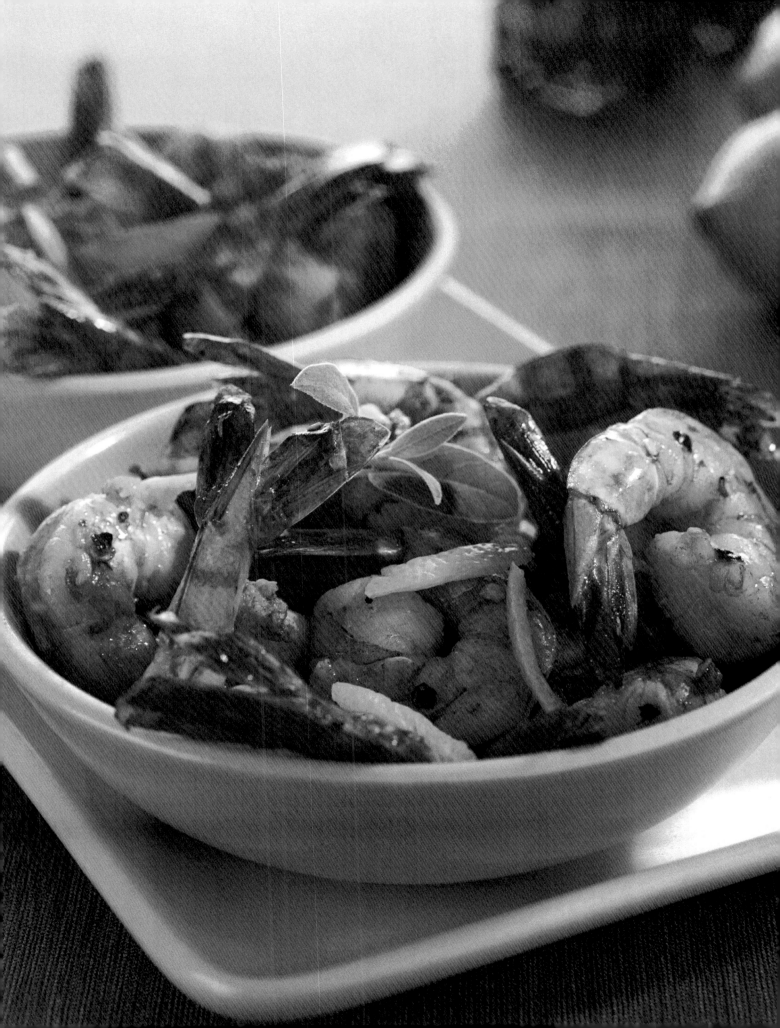

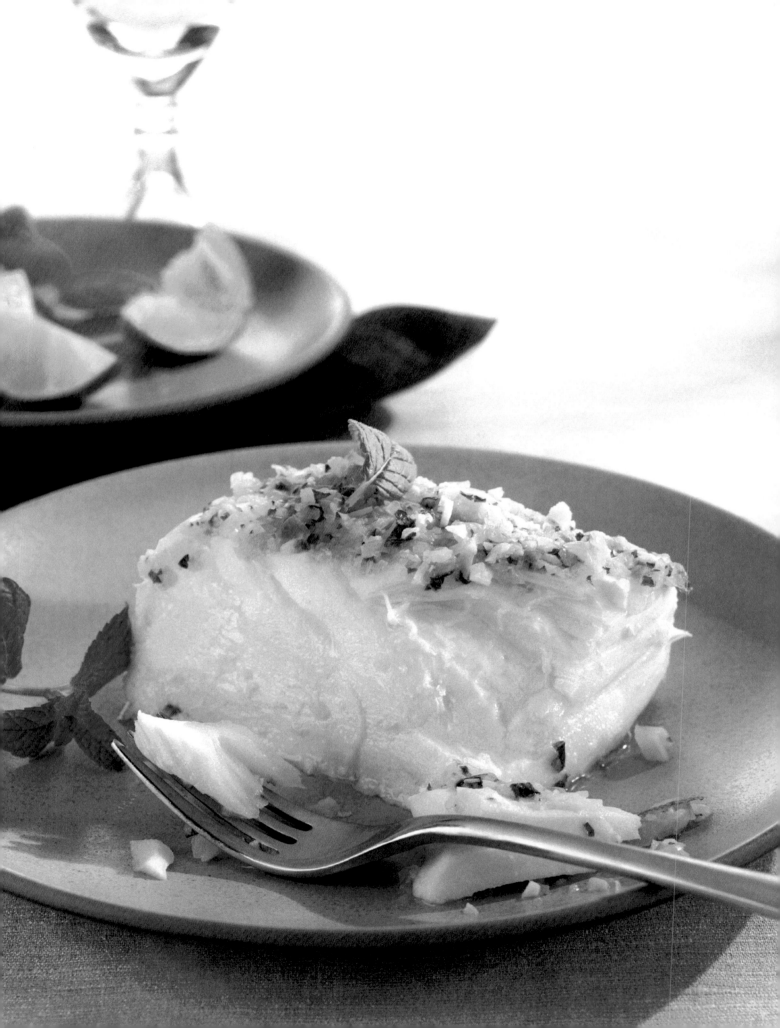

Poached Halibut with Mint Dressing

Serves 2 to 4

Ingredients

1 lb. of filleted halibut, portioned

4 tbsp of lime juice

4 tbsp of lime zest

4 cloves of garlic, minced

1 bunch of shallots

1 bunch of fresh mint, chopped

salt and pepper

Preparation

- Blend the lime juice, lime zest, shallots, and mint in a food processor for 30 seconds.

- Spread the garlic evenly over the fish on a plate.

- Spread the mixture on top of the garlic.

- Season with salt and pepper.

- Pour $1/3$ cup of water into a frying pan and bring to a boil.

- Place the pieces of fish into the boiling water and cover.

- Steam the fish until its layers begin to separate but it is still juicy (approximately 7 to 10 minutes).

Rice Vinegar Shrimp and Cucumbers

Serves 2 to 4

Ingredients

8 cucumbers, peeled and thinly sliced

4 scallions, sliced

⅓ cup of rice vinegar

1 lb. of baby shrimp, cooked

1 tbsp of fennel seeds

Preparation

- Mix all the ingredients in a bowl.
- Refrigerate for an hour before serving.

Courtesy of Janis Kanter

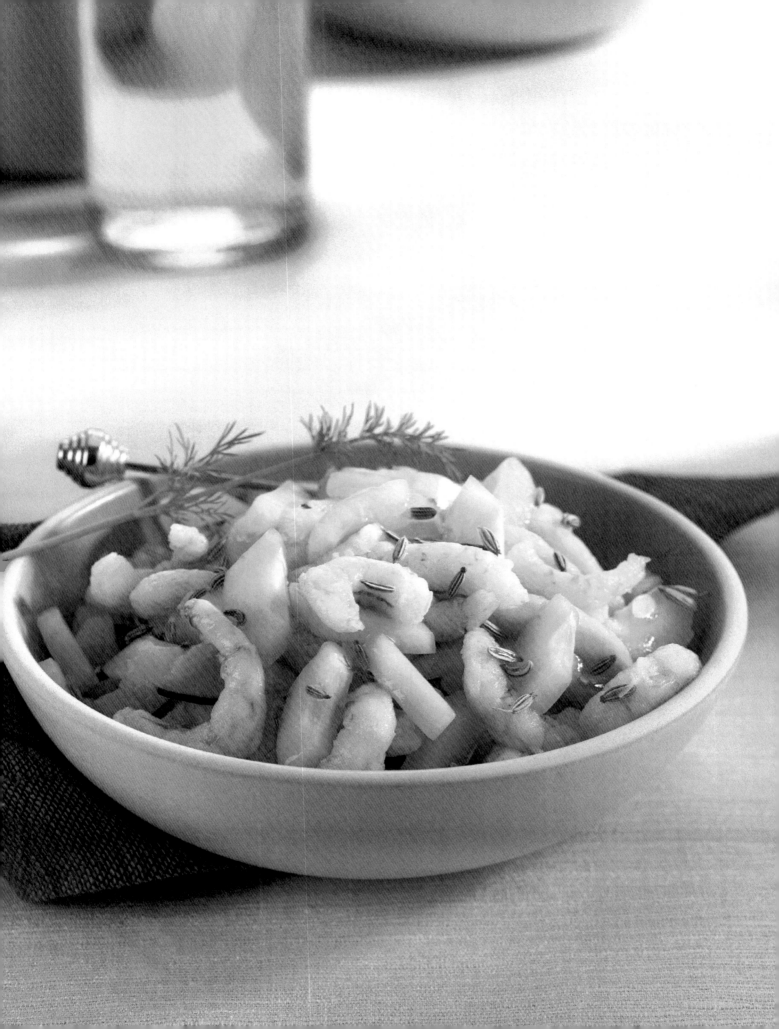

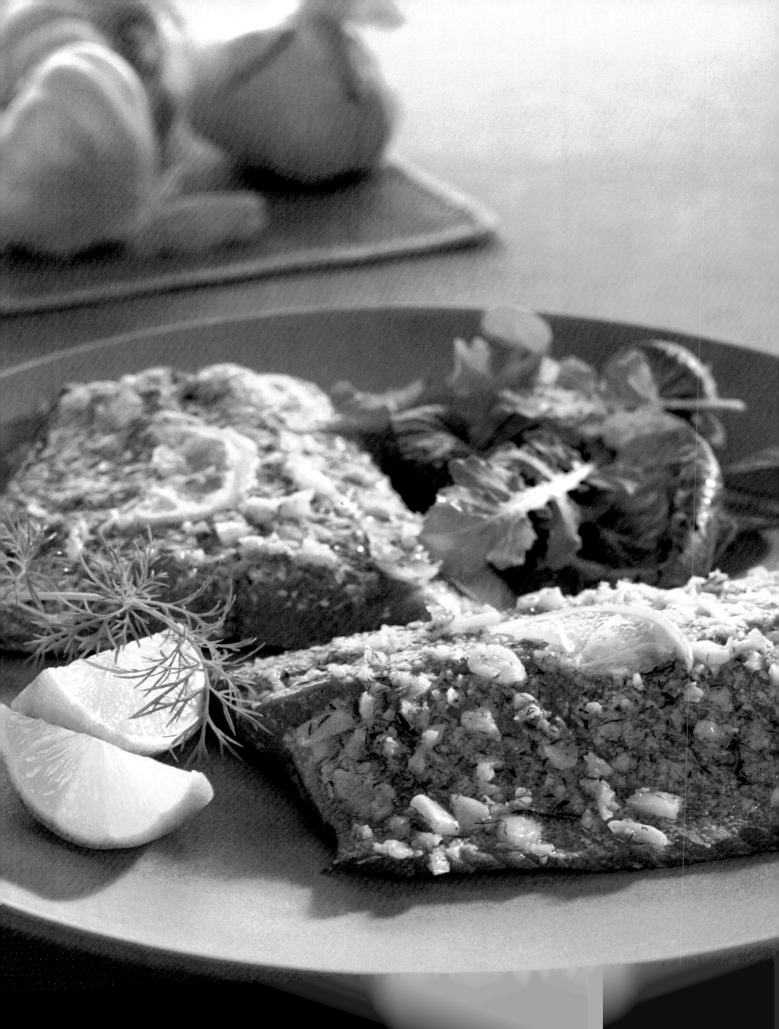

Salmon with Dill Sauce

Serves 2 to 4

Ingredients

2 ½ lbs of fresh wild salmon fillet

1 bunch of fresh dill

5 cloves of garlic, minced

3 lemons, sliced

2 tsp of olive oil

garlic salt

pepper

Preparation

- Blend the dill, garlic, and olive oil into a paste in a food processor.
- Place the salmon on a sheet of aluminum foil.
- Sprinkle the garlic salt and pepper on the salmon.
- Spread the paste on the salmon with a spatula.
- Heat the oven to 350° F.
- Wrap the salmon in the foil and place in the oven for 1 hour.
- Garnish with lemon slices.
- Serve hot or cold.

Spiced Tuna

Serves 2 to 4

Ingredients

1 lb. of tuna

1 tbsp of fennel seeds

1 tbsp of cumin seeds

1 tbsp of sesame seeds

2 tbsp of coriander seeds

¼ cup of fresh ginger, coarsely chopped

5 cloves of garlic, crushed

4 tbsp of extra virgin olive oil

salt

red pepper flakes

Preparation

- Position a rack on a rimmed baking sheet in the center of the oven and preheat to 450º F.

- Grind all the spices in a food processor until the mixture is finely chopped (about 30 seconds).

- Pour 3 tbsp of the olive oil into the food processor and grind again, stopping to scrape down the sides until the mixture forms a paste (about 20 seconds).

- Rub 1 tbsp of olive oil on the tuna.

- Sprinkle 2 tbsp of salt evenly over the tuna.

- Spread the spice paste onto the tuna with your hands.

- Place the tuna on the rack.

- Roast the tuna to taste (15 to 18 minutes for medium rare).

Courtesy of Alheli Maahs

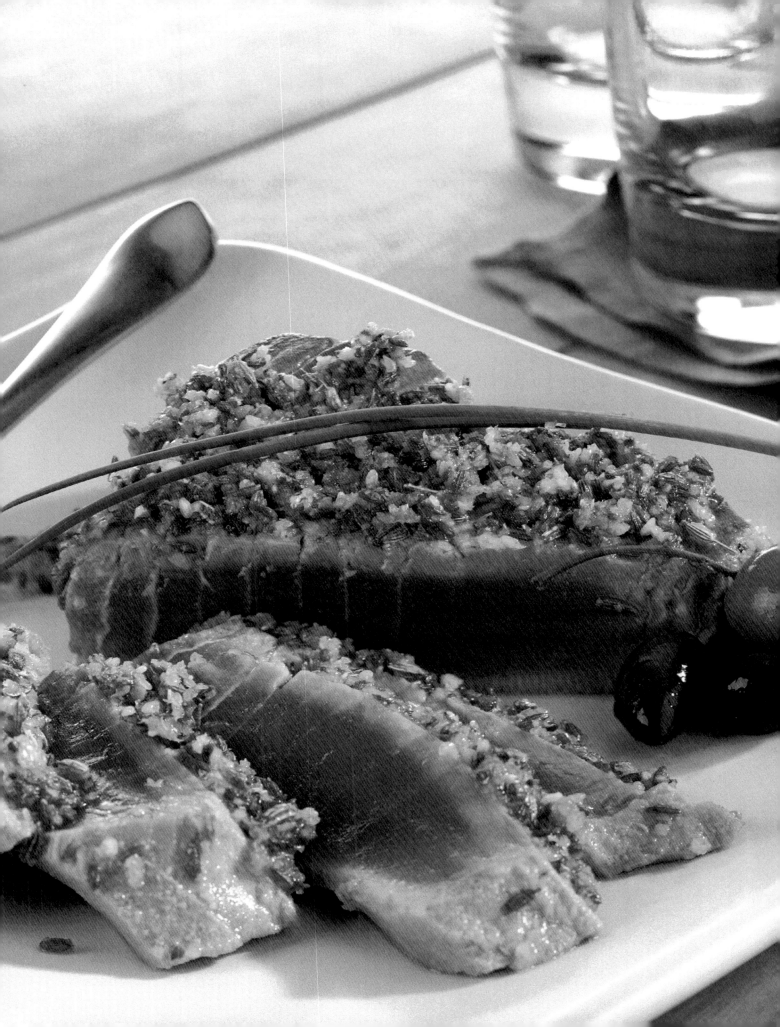

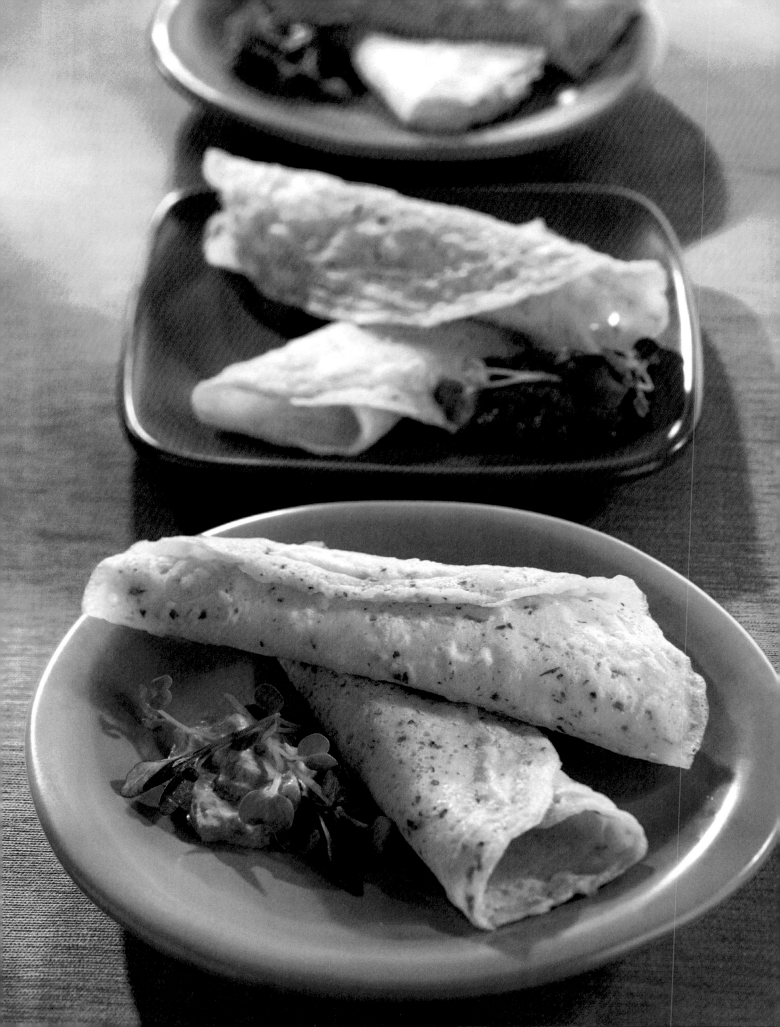

Lentil Crepes

Serves 1 to 2

Ingredients

½ cup lentil (mung dal) flour

1 cup water

½ inch cube ginger (optional)

1 tbsp finely chopped cilantro

canola oil for pan-frying

salt to taste

Preparation

- Blend lentil flour, water, salt, cilantro and ginger in the blender. Add water if needed to get a crepe batter consistency.

- Scoop on to an oiled, flat crepe pan, and spread it thin like a crepe.

- Once there are bubbles on the top, flip, and cook the other side.

- Serve with a tomato or cilantro chutney or top with bananas for kids.

Courtesy of Komal Shah

Paneer Jalfrezie

Serves 2 to 4

Ingredients

¹/₂ bell pepper

¹/₂ onion

10 oz. paneer* or firm tofu

4 oz. organic canned tomato sauce

2 tbsp canola oil

¹/₂ tsp turmeric

¹/₂ tsp garam masala or curry powder

2 tsp coriander powder

¹/₂ tsp cumin seeds

2 tsp sugar

salt to taste

*Paneer is Indian Farmer cheese available in the refrigerated section of Indian stores. For a vegan recipe, you can substitute with firm tofu.

Preparation

- Chop the onion and bell-pepper in thin long strips

- Cut the paneer or tofu into about 2 x ½ x ½ inch strips

- Heat the oil in a flat pan and add cumin seeds

- When the seeds sizzle, turn down the heat to low, and add the onions and bell peppers.

- Add salt, turmeric, garam masala, coriander powder, and sugar

- Sauté the onions and peppers for 2 minutes

- Add tomato sauce and let it simmer for 2 minutes.

- Add paneer or tofu, stirring very gently until the they are coated with gravy

- Let simmer for 2-3 more minutes on low heat and enjoy!

Courtesy of Komal Shah

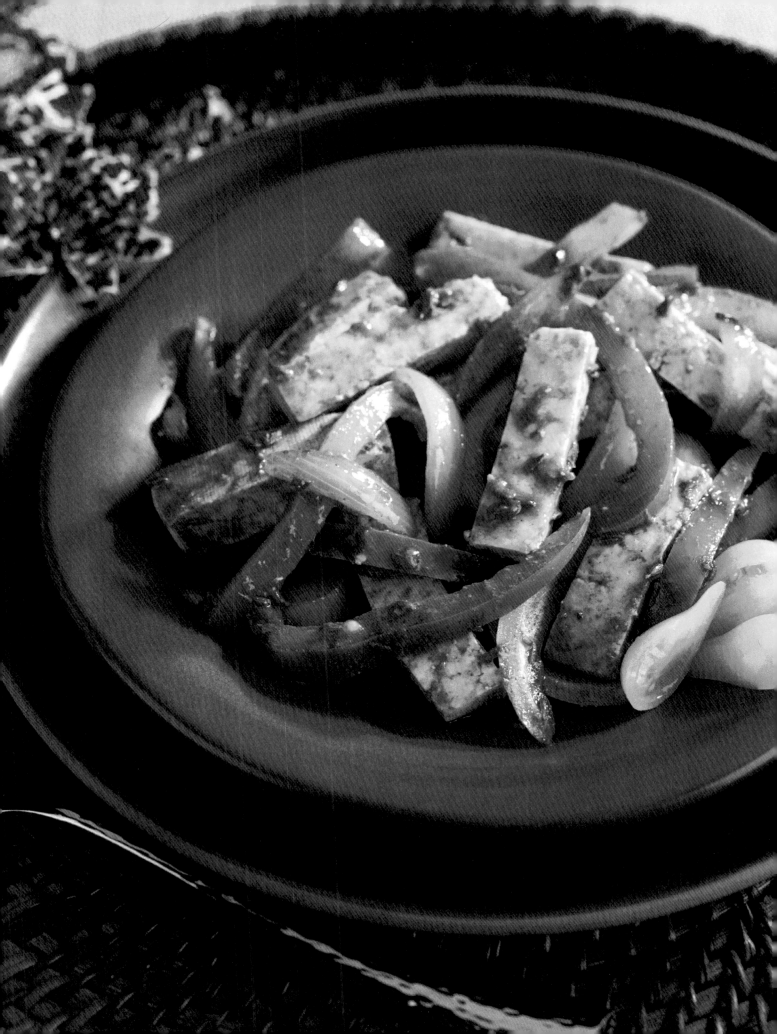

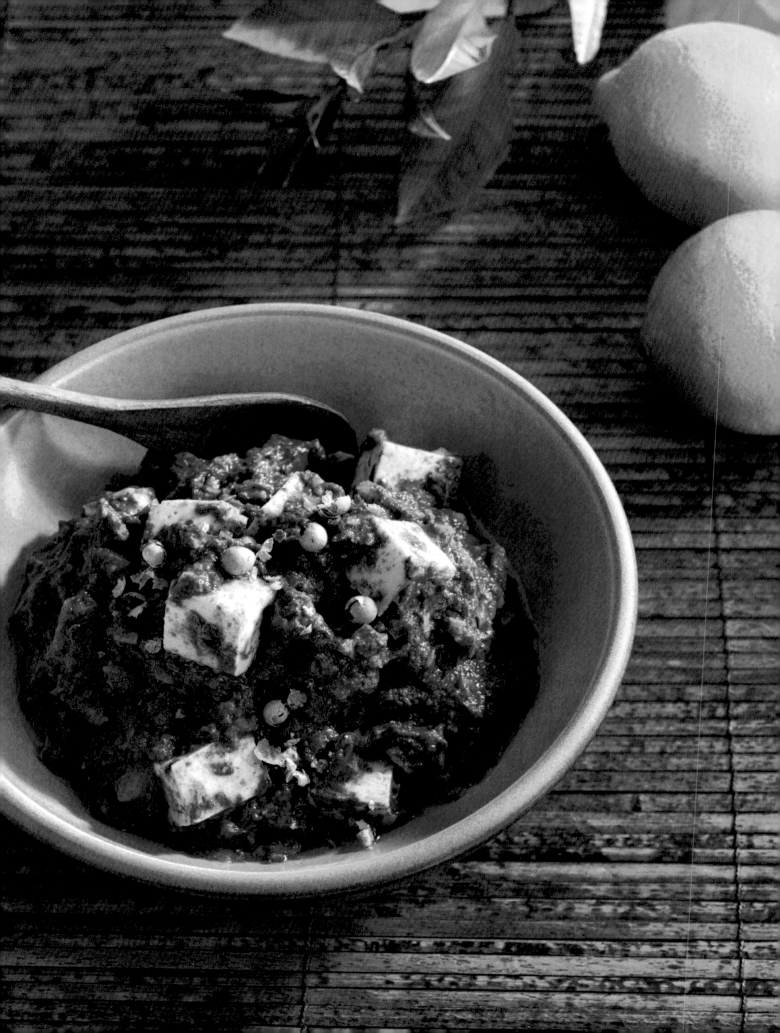

Palak Paneer

Serves 2 to 4

Ingredients

1 lb. baby spinach (organic)

8 oz. paneer or firm tofu (cut into ½ inch cubes)

2 onions

1 inch cube ginger

1 tsp cumin seeds

2 tbsp canola oil

½ tsp turmeric

1 tsp garam masala (or curry powder)

salt to taste

2 tsp coriander powder

lemon juice from ½ lemon

Preparation

- Puree the onions and ginger in a blender.

- Heat oil in a pot, and add cumin seeds.

- When the cumin seeds sizzle, add the onion puree, and let it cook for 10-15 minutes on low heat, stirring occasionally.

- Wash spinach and microwave in a large container with 1 cup of water for 7 minutes.

- Blend into a puree after the spinach is cooked. Add more water if needed to ensure a gravy consistency.

- Add the spinach to the onion gravy.

- Add garam masala, coriander powder, salt, lemon juice, and let simmer for 10 minutes.

- Add tofu or paneer cubes, simmer for 2 more minutes and serve.

Courtesy of Komal Shah

Lentil Stew

Serves 1 to 2

Ingredients

$^1/_2$ onion

1 inch cube ginger

1 clove garlic

1 cup french lentils

2 tbsp canola oil

$^1/_2$ tsp cumin seeds

$^1/_2$ lemon juiced

salt to taste

$^1/_2$ garam masala
(or $^1/_2$ tsp curry powder)

cilantro chopped
(optional)

Preparation

• Boil or pressure cook lentils in salty water
($^1/_2$ tsp salt, 3 cups water). When they are tender to
the touch, set aside.

• Peel and puree onion, garlic, and ginger in a blender.

• Heat the oil in a pot and add cumin seeds.

• When the cumin seeds sizzle, turn the heat low, and
add the onion-ginger-garlic paste.

• Cook for about 5-7 minutes, until the onion puree
looks pinkish or appears cooked.

• Add the cooked lentils with the remaining water.

• Add garam masala and lemon juice. Add salt and
additional water to taste.

• Let the lentils cook for about 15 minutes.

• Sprinkle some chopped cilantro for a fresh flavor.

Courtesy of Komal Shah

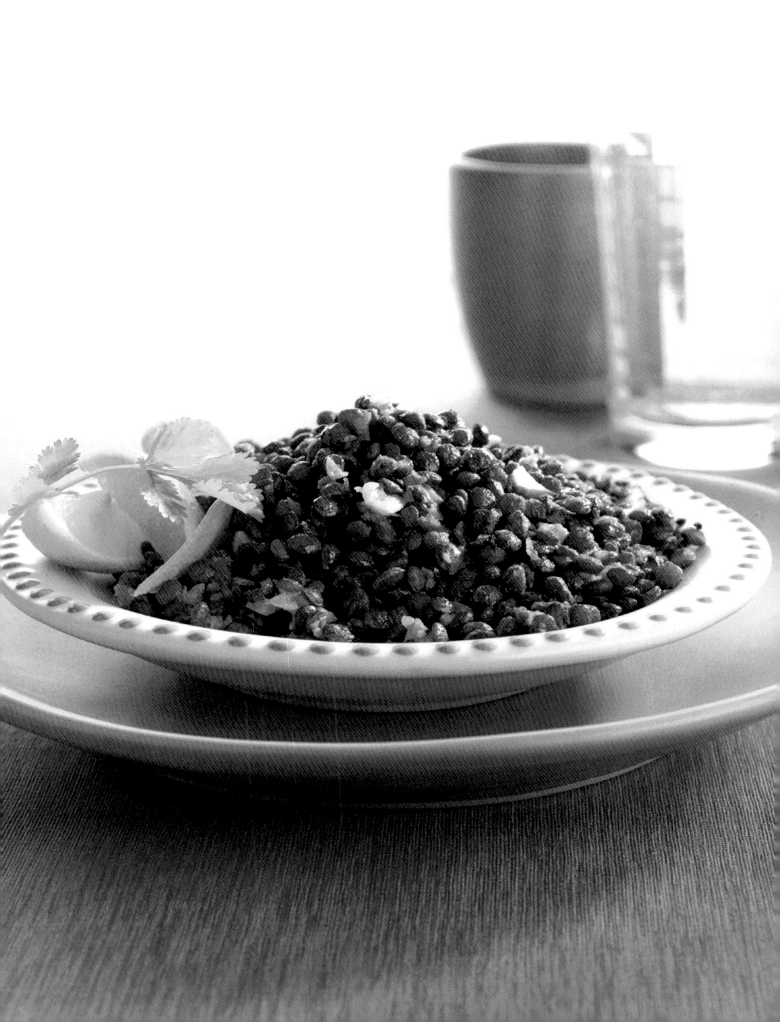

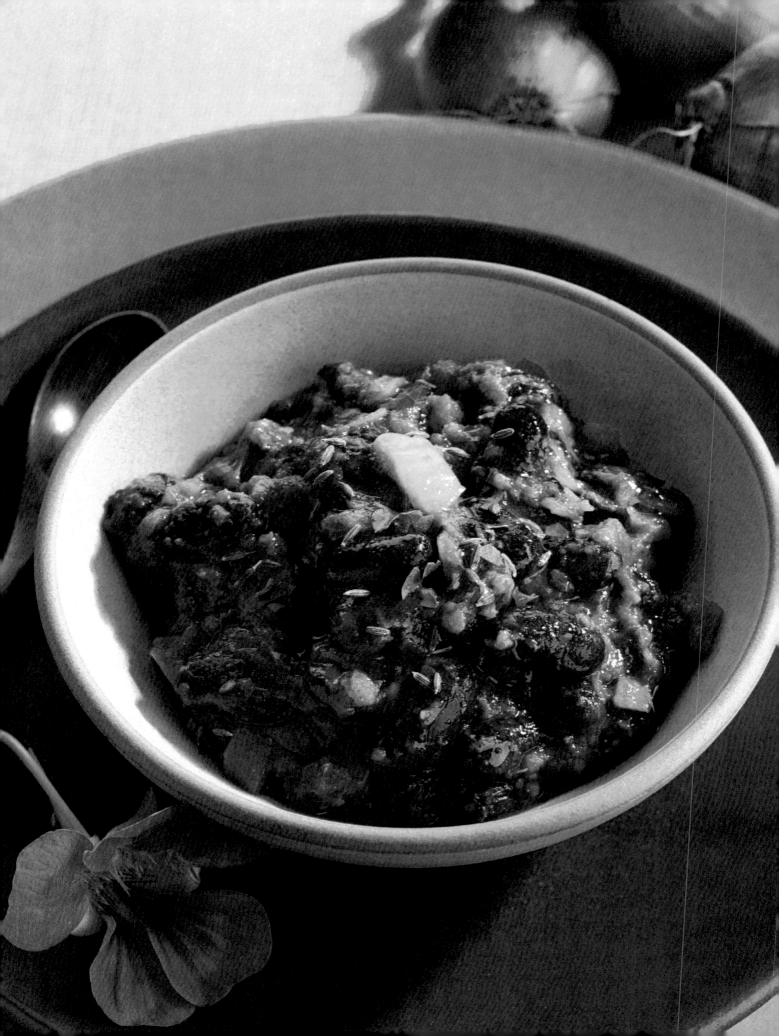

Rajma

Serves 2 to 4

Ingredients

2 onions

1 inch cube ginger

5 cloves garlic

**Two 15 oz. organic
canned kidney beans**

2 tbsp canola oil

1/2 tsp cumin seeds

**5 oz. organic canned
tomato sauce**

**1/2 tsp garam masala
  (or 1/2 tsp curry powder)**

1/4 tsp turmeric

salt to taste

Preparation

- Wash and drain the kidney beans, and set aside.

- Peel and puree onion, garlic, and ginger in a blender.

- Heat the oil in a pot, and add cumin seeds.

- When the cumin seeds sizzle, turn the heat low, and add the onion-ginger-garlic paste.

- Cook for about 10 minutes on low heat stirring occasionally until the onion puree looks pinkish or appears cooked.

- Add the tomato sauce, turmeric, garam masala, and let it simmer for 5 minutes.

- Add the kidney beans.

- Add salt and additional water to taste.

- Let the kidney beans cook for about 15 minutes.

Courtesy of Komal Shah

Asparagus with Shitake Mushrooms

Serves 1 to 2

Ingredients

1 bunch of asparagus

1 lb. of shitake mushrooms

¹⁄₈ cup of roasted pine nuts

chicken broth

Girard's balsamic vinaigrette salad dressing (fat-free)

Preparation

- Steam the asparagus.

- Slice the mushrooms.

- Brown the mushrooms in a frying pan.

- Add fat-free chicken broth to the pan to keep the mushrooms from sticking.

- Brown the pine nuts in a separate pan.

- Place the mushrooms on top of the asparagus.

- Add the salad dressing sparingly.

- Top with pine nuts.

Courtesy of Judy Kiel

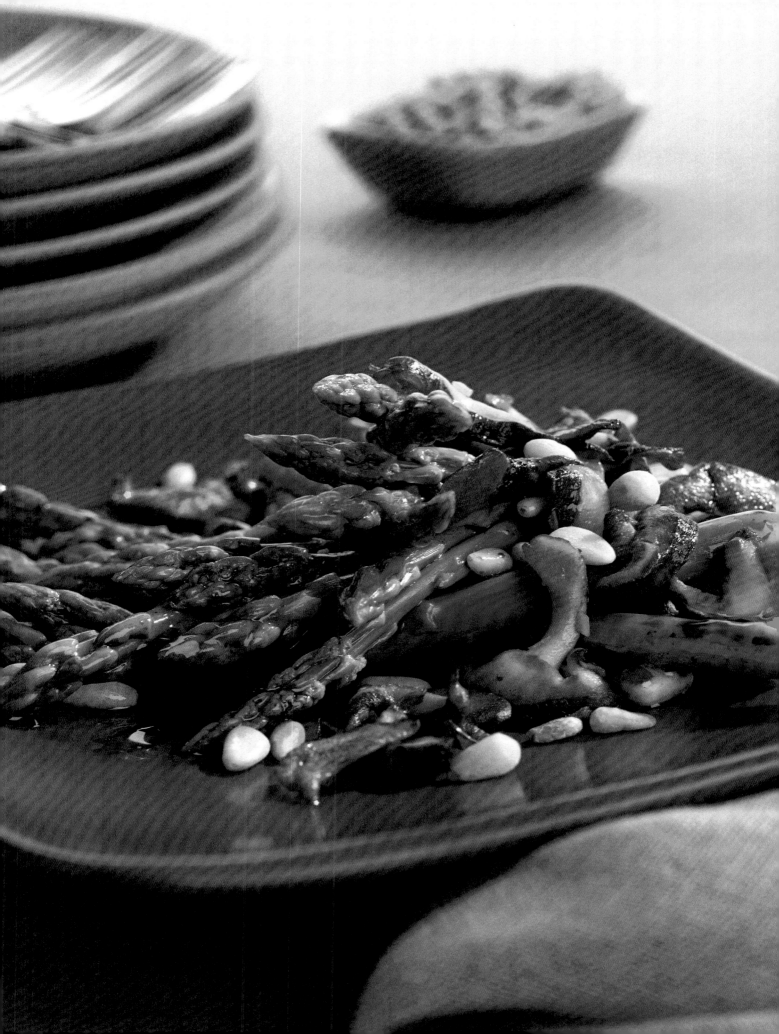

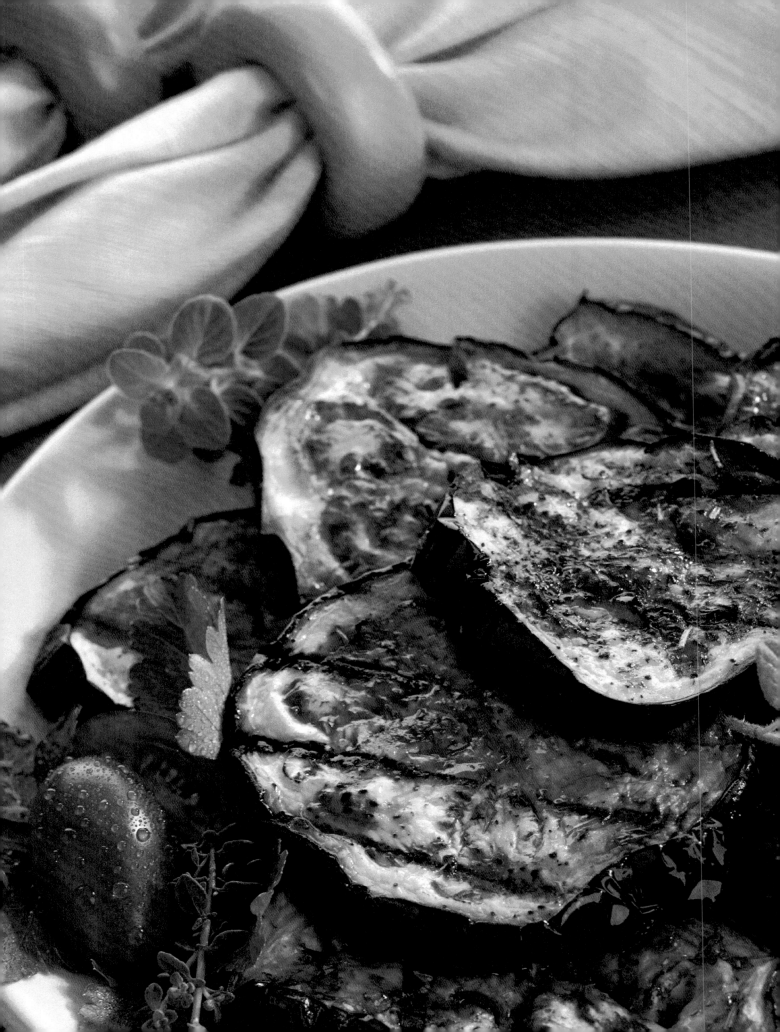

Broiled Eggplant with Garlic and Italian Seasoning

Serves 1 to 2

Ingredients

1 eggplant

5 cloves of garlic, crushed

1 tbsp of olive oil (or nonstick spray)

Italian seasoning

salt and pepper to taste

Preparation

- Slice the eggplant into quarter-inch rounds.

- Thinly spread olive oil on a cookie sheet (or use a nonstick spray).

- Place the eggplant slices on the cookie sheet.

- Sprinkle the garlic on the slices.

- Add the Italian seasoning, salt, and pepper to taste.

- Place the cookie sheet in a broiler and cook for about 4 minutes at 450º F until the eggplant is brown on top.

- Remove the cookie sheet from the broiler. Flip over the slices. Return the cookie sheet to the broiler, and again cook until the eggplant is brown.

Courtesy of Judy Kiel

European Butter Lettuce Salad

Serves 1 to 2

Ingredients

2 cups of butter lettuce, hand shredded

1 European cucumber, sliced

2 tomatoes, quartered

1 bunch of radishes, sliced

1 yellow pepper, sliced

1 bunch of scallions, chopped

Dressing

1 bunch of dill, chopped

¼ cup of organic apple cider vinegar, unfiltered

4 tbsp of rice wine vinegar

2 tbsp of olive oil

salt and pepper

Preparation

• Mix all the ingredients gently in a bowl.

• Add salad dressing.

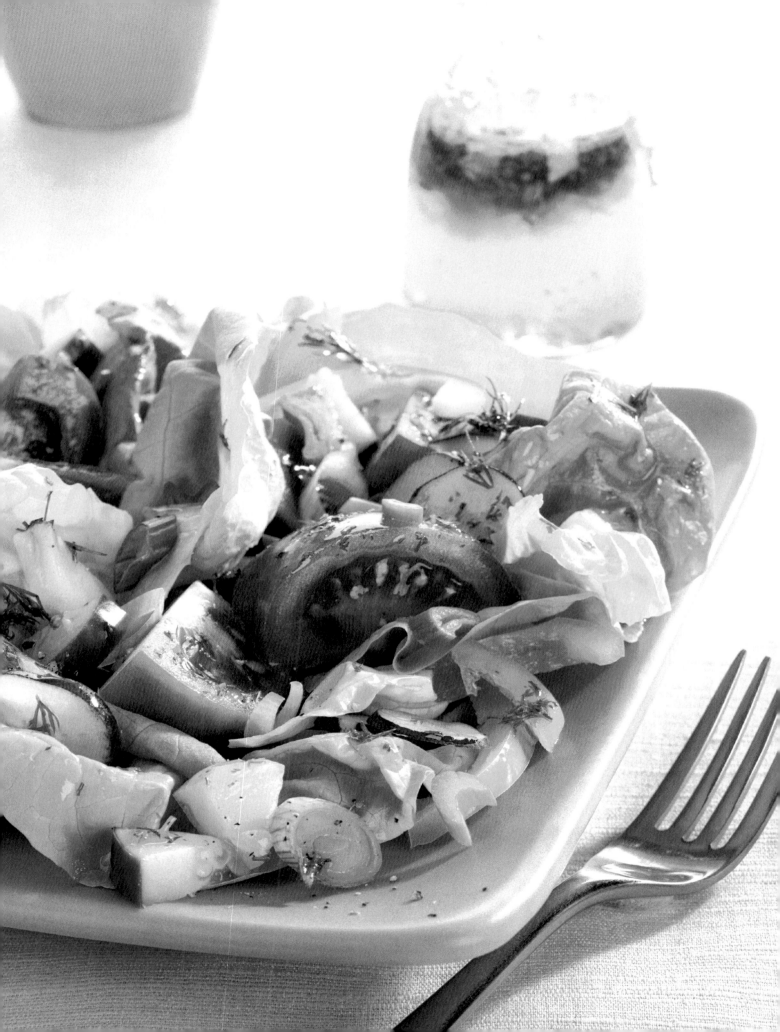

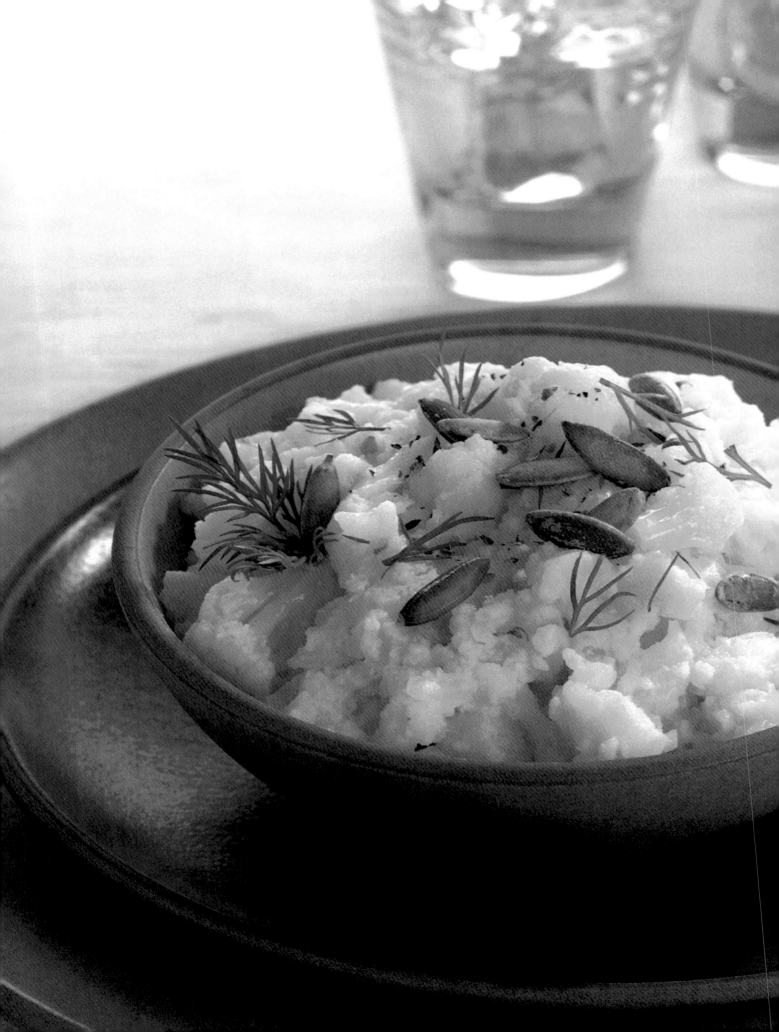

Mashed Cauliflower (Faux Mashed Potatoes)

Serves 1 to 2

Ingredients

1 head of cauliflower

2 cloves of garlic, chopped

$\frac{1}{3}$ can of chicken broth

2 tsp of nonfat milk

salt and pepper

Preparation

- Cut the cauliflower into florets.

- Steam or microwave until the florets are soft (about 8 minutes).

- Place the steamed florets and garlic into a food processor.

- With the machine running, add the broth and milk until the mixture is smooth.

- Place the mixture in a sauce pan.

- Add salt and pepper to taste.

- Simmer on the stove to reheat.

Courtesy of Christy Neidig

Shredded Brussels Sprouts

Serves 1 to 2

Ingredients

2 lbs of Brussels sprouts

1 tbsp of olive oil

2 cloves of garlic, minced

$\frac{1}{3}$ cup of chicken broth

salt and pepper

Preparation

- Cut away the stem ends of each sprout.

- Run the sprouts through a food processor using a slicing blade.

- Heat the olive oil in a nonstick skillet at a medium-high temperature.

- When the oil is hot, add the sprouts and garlic.

- Using a wooden spatula, toss the mixture until it becomes bright green and somewhat soft.

- Add the chicken broth, and allow the sprouts to steam as the liquid evaporates.

- Add salt and pepper to taste.

- Serve hot.

Courtesy of Christy Neidig

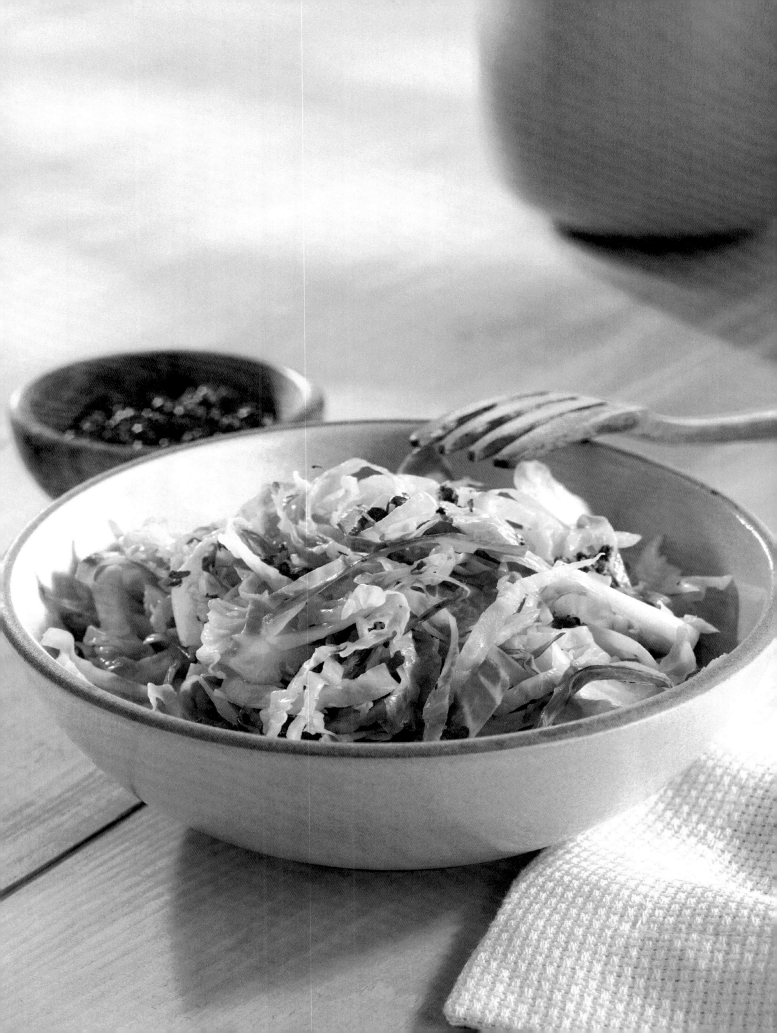

You Can Never Outsmart Your Body

Peter E. Schwab (64-year-old banker)

L osing weight is easy. Keeping it off is hard. I am 64 years old, and for the first 62 years of my life I always had a weight problem. I wasn't obese, but I was overweight enough that I didn't look or feel good. I was also stiff with aches and pains and was starting to feel my age. Interestingly, I never got sick, but I sensed that if I kept going down this path, I was going to become an old man very fast.

I tried every diet in the book. Each worked, and I lost weight. But as soon as I returned to my old eating habits, back came the pounds.

Although I had been jogging for twenty years, forty-five minutes a day, six times a week (and I *loved* every minute of it), it did nothing to keep off my weight. It also did nothing to keep me flexible or get rid of my aches and pains.

Then, one day, I went to lunch with a friend I had known since high school, and I noticed how terrific he looked. I asked him if he had been dieting or working out, and he told me about Jerzy and The Happy Body program. I couldn't get Jerzy's phone number fast enough!

A few days later, as I was driving to my first appointment, I imagined that Jerzy would be a typical California trainer, with a tan and bulging muscles. Boy, was I wrong! The man I met was very special. He was an intellectual, a terrific teacher, and a weightlifting champion, and he had a clear vision of how he wanted to make me youthful.

The first thing he said is that the work was not going to be easy and would take time. Then he told me that jogging was actually the worst thing I could do for my body—that it was one of the fastest ways to age myself. At that point, I almost walked out the door. When he told me that the program would involve lifting weights for thirty minutes every day, I almost walked out the door a second time, because I had always hated weight training. But when he told me that in one year he could help me to have a body that was as strong and flexible as it had been in my twenties, and that he would support me every step of the way, I decided to put myself in his hands.

So, I stopped jogging and, after a month or so, started to enjoy lifting weights. In fact, I came to love it even more than jogging. My body fat dropped to 16% as I lost 44 pounds of fat and gained 10 pounds of muscle. Best of all, I felt great.

[CONTINUED ON NEXT PAGE]

Then, after maintaining the program on my own for a while, I thought I could outsmart my body by continuing the exercises while discontinuing The Happy Body food plan. In no time, I had all the pounds back. When I went to see Jerzy again, instead of criticizing me, he explained all the reasons I was having such a hard time staying with the food plan. As I was talking to him, the light suddenly went on in my head: This was not a diet, it was a lifestyle change, and I had to make it part of my life. Once I made that commitment, I appreciated what Jerzy had been saying all along: "You cannot buy or be given youthfulness. You have to earn it."

Now I understand that you can never outsmart your body. If you want it to be happy, you must have a perfect balance between how you eat and how you exercise.

INGREDIENTS FOR A BETTER YOU

Holding this book in your hands means that you, like our clients, aspire to a youthful and graceful lifestyle. After reading The Happy Body book you know about the happy body. In order to become a happy body, you need to go back to Part 2, the section that outlines the practice, and begin your journey. You will find that there are some steps that are easy and others that are challenging.

If you find yourself thinking it will be difficult, tell yourself, *I will embrace it. It may take a long time, but I will keep doing until I get it. I do not have enough energy, but if I get stronger and lose weight I will have more energy. I do not believe it will work, but I will test it by doing everything that the program requires.* Develop a positive and constructive attitude. It will lead to the right decisions to move you forward.

The Happy Body program is based on solid and meaningful truths. One of them is learning and embracing how much is enough. Once Jerzy explained to Billy Robertson, a car racer and a client, that it is not only wise to live between too much and too little, but it is also the fastest and most safe way to improve. Billy responded, "It is exactly like that in car racing. When I hear my car tires sliding, I know that my car is slowing down because it is losing traction. I have to correct this by releasing the accelerator. On the other hand, if I don't hear sliding tires, I am driving too slowly. I adjust between the two extremes all during a race. The only way to know enough is to make mistakes, learn from them and make educated guesses to narrow the gap between too much and too little."

You do not need any special talent or skill in order to make the changes you desire. What you do need is to persevere and to enjoy the journey. Cherish every meal. Take pleasure with every movement and breath when you exercise. When listening to the meditation tape be grateful for all your efforts. At the end of the day, take the time to remind yourself that the pursuit of health is worthwhile, that it is within your reach and that gradually small improvements accumulate. These practices will nurture and make a better you.

Buettner, Dan. *The Blue Zones.* Washington, D.C.: National Geographic, 2008.

Byrne, Phonda. *The Secret.* New York: Arai Books, 2006.

Cambell, T. Colin, and Thomas M. Campbell II. *The China Study.* Dallas: Benbella Books, 2006.

Carson, Rick. *Taming Your Gremlin.* New York: Collins, 2003.

Charan, Ram. *Know-How.* New York: Crown Business, 2007.

Chilton, Floyd H. *Inflammation Nation.* New York: A Fireside Book, 2005.

Chopra, Deepak. *Quantum Healing.* New York: Bantam Books, 1989.

Drechsler, Arthur. *The Weightlifting Encyclopedia.* Whitestone: A Is A Communications, 1998.

Dyer, Dr. Wayne W. *Excuses Begone!* Carlsbad: Hay House, Inc, 2009.

—. *Change Your Thoughts Change Your Life.* Carlsbad: Hay House, 2007.

Fehér, Tamás. *Olympic Weightlifting.* Budapest: Tamas Strength Sport Libri Publishing House, 2007.

Feldenkrais, Moshe. *The Master Moves.* Capitola: Meta Publications, 1984.

—. *Body Awareness as Healing Therapy.* Berkeley: Somatic Resources, 1997.

Frankl, Viktor E. *Man's Search for Meaning.* New York: Washington Square Press, 1984.

—. *The Doctor and the Soul.* New York: Vintage Books, 1986.

Gilbert, Daniel. *Stumbling on Happiness.* New York: Vintage Books, 2005.

Gladwell, Malcolm. *Blink.* New York: Little, Brown and Company, 2005.

—. *The Tipping Point.* New York: Little, Brown and Company, 2002.

Goldman, Robert, Ronald Klatz and Lisa Berger. *Brain Fitness.* New York: Broadway Books, 1999.

Goodall, Jane. *Harvest for Hope.* New York: Warner Books, 2002.

Hallinan, Joseph T. *Why We Make Mistakes.* New York: Broadway Books, 2009.

Hoffman, Jay. *Physiological Aspects of Sport Training and Performance.* Champaign: Human Kinetics, 2002.

Hyman, Mark. *The UltraMind Solution.* New York: Scribner, 2008.

Jubb, Annie Padden, and David. *Secrets of an Alkaline Body.* Berkeley: North Atlantic Books, 2004.

Kessler, David A. *The End of Overeating.* New York: Rodale, 2009.

Lehler, Jonah. *How We Decide.* New York: Houghton Mifflin Harcourt, 2009.

Loehr, Jim, and Tony Schwartz. *The Power of Full Engagement.* New York: Free Press, 2003.

McGill, Stuart. *Ultimate Back Fitness and Performance.* Waterloo: Wabuno Publishers, 2004.

—. *Lower Back Disorders.* Champaign: Human Kinetics, 2002.

Orlick, Terry. *In Pursuit of Excellence.* Champaign: Leisure Press, 1990.

Pollan, Michael. *In Defense of Food.* New York: The Penguin Press, 2008.

—. *The Omnivore's Dilemma.* New York: The Penguin Press, 2006.

Tolle, Eckhart. *The Power of Now.* Novato: Namaste Publishing, 1999.

Ury, William. *The Power of a Positive No.* New York: Bantam Books, 2007.

FINDING ENOUGH

Finding enough is a constant interaction between doing too much and doing too little. It is a part of any craft and ensures the fastest and safest progress. Making mistakes is part of the learning process. Equally important is maintaining trust that you will succeed just like others before you.

This book is designed as a manual. Our clients find reading testimonies and highlighting meaningful passages in the book is inspiring—it keeps them motivated and positive. Record your daily thoughts, feelings, challenges and solutions in your notebook. By re-reading what you marked and wrote you will discover how you are changing. Page by page, mark by mark, The Happy Body will gradually find a home in you. And when it settles, the book will no longer be necessary. You will know how much is enough—enough food, enough exercise, and enough meditation—for you to become a Happy Body.

After shifting their focus from always seeking more to one in which enough is the goal, our clients become joyful, not only because they are fit and healthy, but also because they are in tune with nature. There is overwhelming gracefulness in living *without waste*.

Index

Page numbers of illustrations appear in italics followed by the letter i.

Page numbers of tables and charts appear in italics followed by the letter t.

Titles of recipes appear in italics.

ABOUT THE AUTHORS

Aniela and Jerzy Gregorek came to the United States from Poland in 1986 as political refugees during the Solidarity Movement. As a professional athlete, Aniela has won five World Weightlifting Championships and established six world records. Jerzy has won four World Weightlifting Championships and established one world record. They have also been professional coaches and personal trainers since coming to this country. In 2000, they founded the UCLA weightlifting team and became its head coaches.

Over the years, they have transformed hundreds of people, from housewives and physicians to athletes and celebrities, who came to them with every conceivable body shape and desire. Some wanted to improve their

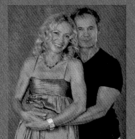

athletic performance; others had never trained before and wanted to lose weight and be attractive; still others just wanted to be able to get down on the floor and play with their grandchildren. But regardless of the words they used to explain why they wanted coaching, there was a clear pattern in their motivations: Everyone wanted to be youthful. Aniela and Jerzy have devoted the last three decades of their lives to finding solutions to this universal goal. In the course of this search, they invented The Happy Body program.

They have both earned MFA degrees in Creative Writing from Norwich University, in Vermont. In their free time, Aniela and Jerzy write poetry and translate poetry both from Polish to English and from English to Polish. Their poetry and translations have appeared in major poetry magazines. Their translation of Josef Baran's *In a Flash* was a finalist for the PEN USA West Literary Award in 2001. The National Endowment for the Arts awarded Jerzy the Literature Fellowship in 2003 to support the translation of selected poems by Maurycy Szymel.

In 2004, after twenty-five years of marriage, Aniela and Jerzy were blessed with the arrival of their precious daughter, Natalie.

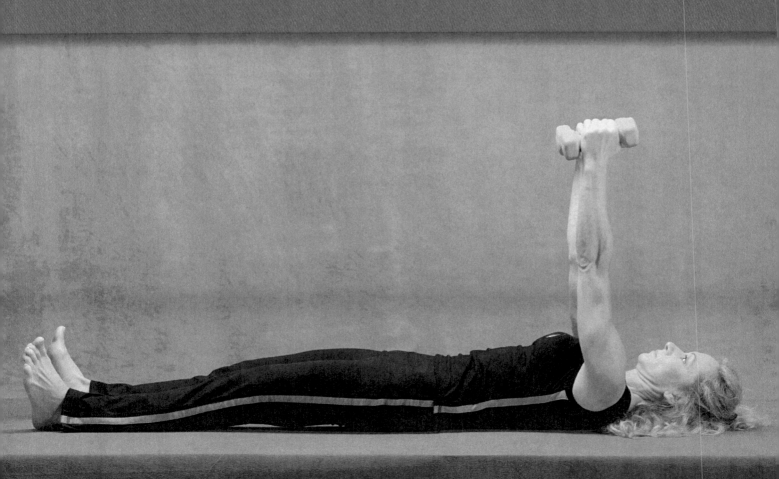

43943308R00173

Made in the USA
San Bernardino, CA
16 July 2019